Modified Rice Bran Arabinoxylan

Sok Cheon Pak • Soo Liang Ooi •
Peter S. Micalos • Mamdooh H. Ghoneum
Editors

Modified Rice Bran Arabinoxylan

Therapeutic Applications in Cancer and Other Diseases

Springer

Editors
Sok Cheon Pak
School of Dentistry and Medical Sciences
Charles Sturt University
Bathurst, NSW, Australia

Soo Liang Ooi
School of Dentistry and Medical Sciences
Charles Sturt University
Bathurst, NSW, Australia

Peter S. Micalos
School of Dentistry and Medical Sciences
Charles Sturt University
Port Macquarie, NSW, Australia

Mamdooh H. Ghoneum
Department of Surgery
Charles Drew University of Medicine & Science
Los Angeles, CA, USA

ISBN 978-981-19-5737-6 ISBN 978-981-19-5735-2 (eBook)
https://doi.org/10.1007/978-981-19-5735-2

This Springer imprint is published by the registered company Springer Nature Singapore Pte Ltd.
The registered company address is: 152 Beach Road, #21-01/04 Gateway East, Singapore 189721, Singapore

Foreword

I have been working with Rice Bran Arabinoxylan Compound (RBAC) for the last 15 years, utilizing it as the treatment in clinical trials and working with individuals who either want to combat a current health challenge or keep the immune system healthy and functional in the first place. Over this time, I have seen countless examples of how this polysaccharide exerts its impressive effects, mostly through improving immune function and/or lowering inflammation according to many biomarkers; the former (improved immune function) being one of the primary mechanisms in preventing chronic disease and the latter (lowering inflammation) being responsible for driving chronic diseases. As I reflect on the voluminous level of information that has been published about RBAC's impressive effects, including that of my own work, I am grateful for the opportunity to have participated in this ongoing and continuing journey of discovery. Truly, the information about RBAC's effects should be spread everywhere so that more people can benefit from it.

To that end, I believe that Dr. Pak and his colleagues have chosen a very worthy cause by writing and editing this book to summarize all of the current information about RBAC in the scientific literature. Unfortunately, lots of beneficial information in the global repository of peer-reviewed journal articles is not easily accessible to the vast number of people, even those in academia who work outside the fields of nutrition and dietary supplementation. I can recount plenty of lectures where I discussed my research findings to learned healthcare professionals who, before hearing me speak, had no knowledge about the health benefits of polysaccharides in general and RBAC specifically. Thus, I congratulate the editorial team for putting together a book that hopefully will help spread the word about the importance of RBAC and its impressive effects.

While the new and unfamiliar events of the last two years (2020–2022) have had acute, lingering, and detrimental effects on billions of people, other problems, such as cancer, did not go away. It may be that more people are now aware of the importance of a healthy and functional immune system, despite not knowing what a T cell is or what a cytokine does, which may also help to bring this book to the forefront with timely information. The editorial team has done an outstanding job of summarizing how RBAC improves overall immune function, lowers inflammation, and helps improve the quality of life for people afflicted with cancer and other common diseases of our era. In addition, this book provides one source for all of this valuable information, as opposed to requiring someone to spend lots of time on PubMed or other search engines looking for all of this information. This summary will appeal to many people who have limited time and focus in today's stressed out, high-strung world. Thus, this book holds promise for educating people who understand the importance of an optimal immune system or how to improve immune function and why RBAC is a key asset to achieving that. For far too long, the benefits of nutrition and dietary supplementation have been either suppressed or relegated to a dark corner, missing the opportunity to help professionals and laypeople. I believe that the world should know how beneficial RBAC is for achieving and maintaining optimal health, and this book will help to advance that mission. My congratulations to the editorial team for a job well done!

Department of Psychiatry and Behavioral Sciences,
University of Miami Miller School of Medicine,
Miami, FL, USA

John E. Lewis

Preface

Rice bran has been touted as the next big superfood by the popular media due to its high nutritional value and enormous potential for improving health and well-being. This book looks at a modified rice bran extract product called Rice Bran Arabinoxylan Compound, also known as RBAC, MGN-3, or commercially as Biobran. RBAC has shown significant potential for treating cancer and improving the immune health of humans in a variety of medical conditions, and has proven to be more than a temporary news fad. RBAC has been tested in clinical trials for two decades, over which time there has been a steady growth of evidence that supports its position as a substantially beneficial health product.

Our editors started writing the first systematic review article of RBAC in 2018, where we found RBAC to be a complementary therapy for conventional cancer treatment. In 2021, we published a narrative review with an expanded scope covering RBAC's health-promoting properties and clinical applications. Due to the exponential interest in the potential effectiveness of RBAC as a dietary supplement for immune improvement and disease prevention, we have solicited manuscripts from leading RBAC experts in order to write this book, *Modified Rice Bran Arabinoxylan: Therapeutic Applications in Cancer and Other Diseases*. Contributions from experts around the world with a range of research backgrounds have all come to the conclusion—RBAC is a powerful product for improving immune health. Using available primary literature, the authors have collated, interpreted, and synthesized the best and most relevant evidence for the interested public as well as well-trained clinicians.

In particular, this book highlights the effect of RBAC on cancer, a very damaging disease that is a critical health concern of the modern era. There are now many clinical results showing the potential benefits of RBAC in the management of cancer. Astute readers will notice that utmost importance is placed on therapeutic applications of RBAC in cancer. Part I introduces RBAC by detailing its relationship to dietary fibers, chemical composition, and production. Part II details RBAC's therapeutic properties, specifically its enhancement of natural killer cell activity and its immunomodulatory, antioxidant, antiangiogenesis, antiproliferative, and anti-inflammatory effects. Part III then focuses specifically on the therapeutic applications of RBAC for treating cancer, while Part IV details its use for a variety of additional medical conditions such as chronic micro-inflammation, HIV, and hepatitis.

This first edition also reports on preliminary findings where RBAC has been demonstrated to be a strategy for treating a variety of medical conditions; at the same time, underlying theories are presented as to why these results encourage the use of RBAC in preclinical studies. With continuing scientific and medical studies and a better understanding of the mechanisms by which this unique biological response modifier improves immune health, we hope that future editions of the book can provide an even deeper understanding and appreciation of RBAC.

We would like to thank all the chapter authors for their contributions and give special thanks to our publisher, Springer Nature, for this opportunity to publish evidence-based data on RBAC and its therapeutic effects. The collected chapters represent the most up-to-date understanding and findings on RBAC. We sincerely hope that this book will help increase the potential for RBAC to confer health benefits to all those in need.

Bathurst, NSW, Australia — Sok Cheon Pak
Bathurst, NSW, Australia — Soo Liang Ooi
Port Macquarie, NSW, Australia — Peter S. Micalos
Los Angeles, CA, USA — Mamdooh H. Ghoneum

Acknowledgments

For this first edition, we searched across the globe for potential contributors at the forefront of Biobran research. Not only did we successfully find a premiere group of contributors, but we found a group of fascinating people with a diverse range of backgrounds and knowledge. Some of the contributors are research academics, others are university scholars teaching in postgraduate programs, and others are clinicians with significant clinical experience. Each contributor has been very enthusiastic about Biobran, and they have been equally enthusiastic about summarizing and synthesizing the research evidence for Biobran's therapeutic applications into the book you find before you now. Their dedication, tenacity, and passion have been integral to this work, and they have humbled us with their support and their sacrifice of time to make this book possible.

We would also like to thank John Lewis, Terry Golombick, Garth Harris, Daniel Baden, Nori Shirai, and Kentaro Ninomiya for their unwavering support for our vision of an edited book dedicated to evidence-based applications of Biobran.

Finally, we would like to thank the team at Springer Nature for their support and encouragement, in particular Lenold Esithor, for his energy and coordination in the publication of this book.

Contents

Editors and Contributors

About the Editors

Sok Cheon Pak has taught and researched at Charles Sturt University in Australia since 2007. His expertise has been in the field of complementary medicine and has become recognized nationally and internationally through ongoing external research collaborations. His area of interest relates specifically to introducing evidence-based practice to complementary medicine research and practice. This has been based on laboratory experiments incorporating modern medical technologies to identify and evidence the underlying rationale for prescribing therapeutic substances for treatment. Over the years, his principal focus has been on the experimental/clinical application of bee venom to human diseases. The following are two examples of where his research related to bee venom has been acknowledged: (a) His research has been recognized by an invitation from the publishing company Springer to write two chapters on "Chemical Composition of Bee Venom" and "Health Benefits and Uses in Medicine of Bee Venom" for the publication of a book entitled *Bee products: chemical and biological properties*. This invitation is directly related to his research on honeybee venom, focusing on health benefits and uses in medicine. (b) He was appointed as the Guest Editor of a Special Issue on "Bee and wasp venoms: biological characteristics and therapeutic application" for a reputed journal. He currently leads and guides research into nutraceuticals to provide relevant and impactful clinical applications.

Soo Liang Ooi is a nutritionist and naturopath with clinical experience in Australia and Singapore. He holds a BHSc degree from Charles Sturt University, a MBA degree from the National University of Singapore, and a MMath degree from the University of Waterloo in Canada. Soo Liang Ooi is currently pursuing his PhD study in the School of Dentistry and Medical Sciences at Charles Sturt University. His research topic focuses on understanding the immunomodulating properties of rice bran arabinoxylan compound and its effects on the quality of life of cancer patients. His research interests lie in evidence-based complementary medicine, nutritional medicine, naturopathy, herbal medicine, meditation, and integrative cancer therapies. As an avid academic writer, Soo Liang published extensively in major peer-reviewed integrative and complementary medicine journals. He received a nomination for the prestigious Elsevier Atlas award in 2017 for his work on "Transcendental meditation for lowering blood pressure: An overview of systematic reviews and meta-analyses." He is also a co-editor of the Special Issue books on *Health Benefits of Meditation and Nutraceuticals in Immune Function.*

Peter S. Micalos is a teaching-research academic at Charles Sturt University, Australia. Peter commenced teaching and researching exercise and sports science in 1997. In 2012, Peter transferred to the School of Biomedical Sciences to align his PhD studies on pain and exercise with teaching and research in biomedicine. Over this period, Peter has published several research articles and scientific papers in human health, exercise, pain, chronic pain, acupuncture, and complementary medicine. His research has included assessing human physical performance, respiratory and metabolic responses to exercise, pain threshold, spinal nociceptive reflexes, somatosensory evoked potentials, and brain tomography using functional magnetic resonance imaging (fMRI). Peter has presented at national and international research conferences and has supervised several Honors, Masters, and PhD research students.

Mamdooh H. Ghoneum is an internationally recognized expert and pioneer in cancer immunotherapy whose work over the past 30 years has fostered a fundamental paradigm shift from using chemotherapy as a mainstay for cancer treatment toward using natural agents that exert anticancer activity. He has revolutionized the field of cancer immunotherapy by introducing several unique, nontoxic biological response modifiers (BRMs), including arabinoxylan rice bran (MGN-3/Biobran), gross thymic extract (Thymax), and nanodiamond and nanoplatinum particles. These unique BRMs are manufactured using cutting-edge technology and activate the immune system to kill cancer cells and sensitize cancer cells to chemotherapy. The results of his research are currently being applied in major clinical trials all over the world.

John E. Lewis, Ph.D., is past full-time and current Voluntary Associate Professor in the Department of Psychiatry and Behavioral Sciences at the University of Miami Miller School of Medicine and the Founder and President of Dr Lewis Nutrition™ (https://www.drlewisnutrition.com/). He is a Diplomate, Faculty Member, and Advisor of the Medical Wellness Association. He has been the principal investigator of over 30 different studies in his research career, including the clinical trials using RBAC on healthy adults and patients with HIV and non-alcoholic fatty liver disease.

Contributors

Jason Ashworth, PhD Department of Life Sciences, Manchester Metropolitan University, Manchester, UK

Romulo Jacinto S. de Villa, MD PhD National Kidney and Transplant Institute, Quezon City, Metro Manila, Philippines

Yukari Egashira, PhD Laboratory of Food and Nutrition, Division of Applied Biochemistry, Graduate School of Horticulture, Chiba University, Matsudo, Chiba, Japan

Yuzo Endo, MD PhD Hamamatsu University School of Medicine, Hamamatsu, Japan

Jerickson Abbie S. Flores, MD Department of Radiotherapy, Jose R. Reyes Memorial Medical Center, Manila, Philippines

Mamdooh H. Ghoneum, DSc Department of Surgery, Charles R. Drew University of Medicine and Science, Los Angeles, CA, USA

Tibor Hajtó, Prof. Dr. habil. Medical University Pécs, Törökbálint, Hungary

Jayani Kulathunga, PhD candidate Cereal Science Graduate Program, Department of Plant Sciences, North Dakota State University, Fargo, ND, USA

Peter S. Micalos, PhD School of Dentistry & Medical Sciences, Charles Sturt University, Port Macquarie, NSW, Australia

Kentaro Ninomiya, PhD Daiwa Pharmaceutical Co., Ltd., Tokyo, Japan

Soo Liang Ooi, PhD candidate School of Dentistry & Medical Sciences, Charles Sturt University, Bathurst, NSW, Australia

Bahri Ozsisli, PhD Department of Food Engineering, Kahramanmaras Sutcu Imam University, Turkey

Sok Cheon Pak, PhD School of Dentistry & Medical Sciences, Charles Sturt University, Bathurst, NSW, Australia

Jaffar C. Pineda, MD Department of Radiotherapy, Jose R. Reyes Memorial Medical Center, Manila, Philippines

Senay Simsek, PhD Department of Food Science, Whistler Center for Carbohydrate Research, Purdue University, West Lafayette, IN, USA

Abbreviations

ADP	Adenosine diphosphate
AGE	Advanced glycation end products
AHCC	Active hexose correlated compound
AIDS	Acquired immunodeficiency syndrome
ALP	Alkaline phosphatase
ALT	Alanine transaminase
APC	Antigen-presenting cell
ART	Antiretroviral therapy
AST	Aspartate transaminase
ATP	Adenosine triphosphate
AX	Arabinoxylan
BLT	Benzyloxycarbonyl-L-lysine thiobenzyl ester
BRM	Biological response modifier
CA	Carbohydrate antigen
CAM	Complementary and alternative medicine
CAT	Catalase
CBH	Corn bran hemicellulose
CD	Cluster of differentiation
CEA	Carcinoembryonic antigen
CFQ	Chalder fatigue questionnaire
CFS	Chronic fatigue syndrome
CNS	Central nervous system
COX	Cyclooxygenase
CRP	C-reactive protein
CT	Computerized tomography
CTC	Circulating tumor cells
CTLA	Cytotoxic T lymphocyte-associated antigen
DAMP	Damage-associated molecular pattern
DC	Dendritic cell
D-GalN	D-galactosamine
DM	Diabetes mellitus
DNA	Deoxyribonucleic acid
EGFR	Epidermal growth factor receptor

ELISA	Enzyme-linked immunosorbent assay
eNOS	Endothelial nitric oxide synthase
EORTC	European Organization for the Research and Treatment of Cancer
FACT-G	Functional Assessment of Cancer Therapy-General
FLD	Fatty liver disease
GFR	Growth factor receptor
GPx	Glutathione peroxidase
HBV	Hepatitis B virus
HCC	Hepatocellular carcinoma
HCl	Hydrochloric acid
HCV	Hepatitis C virus
HIV	Human immunodeficiency virus
HPV	Human papillomavirus
HRB	Hydrolyzed rice bran
IBS	Irritable bowel syndrome
ICAM-1	Intercellular adhesion molecule 1
IFN	Interferon
Ig	Immunoglobulin
IL	Interleukin
iNOS	Inducible nitric oxide synthase
JAK2	Janus kinase 2
JNK	c-Jun N-terminal kinase
LAK	Lymphokine-activated killer
LDL	Low-density lipoprotein
LMW	Low molecular weight
LPS	Lipopolysaccharide
LTB4	Leukotriene B4
MAPK	Mitogen-activated protein kinase
MEK	Mitogen-activated extracellular signal regulated kinase
MHC-I	Major histocompatibility complex I
MICA/B	MHC class-I chain related A and B
MIP-2	Macrophage inflammatory protein 2
MNC	Mononuclear cell
mPGES-1	Microsomal prostaglandin E synthase 1
MR	Magnetic resonance
mRNA	Messenger ribonucleic acid
MVE-2	Maleic anhydride divinyl ether
NA	Not available
NaCl	Sodium chloride
NAFLD	Non-alcoholic fatty liver disease
NaOH	Sodium hydroxide
NF-κB	Nuclear factor kappa B
NK	Natural killer
NKT	Natural killer T
NO	Nitric oxide

NSCLC	Non-small-cell lung cancer
PD-1	Programmed cell death protein 1
PD-L1	Programmed cell death-1 ligand 1
PGE2	Prostaglandin E2
PGIC	Patient global impression of change
PKC	Protein kinase C
PolyICLC	Polyinosinic:polycytidylic acid stabilized with poly-L-lysine
PPR	Pattern recognition receptor
QLQ-C30	Core 30-item quality of life questionnaire
QoL	Quality of life
RA	Rheumatoid arthritis
RB	Rice bran
RBAC	Rice bran arabinoxylan compound
RCT	Randomized controlled trial
rHu	Recombinant human
RNA	Ribonucleic acid
sCAT	Standardized complementary alternative therapies
SGOT	Serum glutamic-oxaloacetic transaminase
SGPT	Serum glutamic pyruvic transaminase
SOD	Superoxide dismutase
STAT3	Signal transducer and activator of transcription 3
Th	Helper T cell
TLR	Toll-like receptor
TNF	Tumor necrosis factor
Treg	Regulatory T cell
ULBP	UL-16 binding protein
UTP	Uridine triphosphate
VEGF	Vascular endothelial growth factor
WEAX	Water-extractable arabinoxylan
WUAX	Water-unextractable arabinoxylan

List of Figures

List of Table

Part I

Introduction

Part I aims at introducing rice bran arabinoxylan compound (RBAC) to the reader by detailing its relationship to dietary fibers, chemical composition, and production.

Introduction to Rice Bran Arabinoxylan Compound

1

Jayani Kulathunga, Bahri Ozsisli, and Senay Simsek

Abstract

The role of non-starch polysaccharides of cereals in health and nutrition has stimulated a wide range of research activities. Arabinoxylans are the major non-starch polysaccharide constituents of cereals, and they are predominantly found in the outer layers of the grain. They are composed of backbone chains of α-(1-4)-linked D-xylopyranosyl residues to which α-L-arabinofuranose units are linked as side chains. Rice bran has been identified as an underutilized source of dietary fiber, and there is a great potential to produce modified/unmodified arabinoxylans as a nutraceutical. The available studies have shown the health beneficial effects of rice bran arabinoxylans such as immunomodulatory, antioxidant, anticarcinogenic, and antiproliferative properties. This introductory book chapter summarizes the available information on rice bran, rice bran dietary fiber, and its relationship to rice bran arabinoxylans and rice bran arabinoxylan structure.

Keywords

Dietary fiber · Nutraceutical · Water extraction · MGN-3 · Biobran

J. Kulathunga
Department of Plant Sciences, Cereal Science Graduate Program, North Dakota State University, Fargo, ND, USA

B. Ozsisli
Department of Food Engineering, Kahramanmaras Sutcu Imam University, Kahramanmaras, Turkey

S. Simsek (✉)
Department of Food Science, Whistler Center for Carbohydrate Research, Purdue University, West Lafa-yette, IN, USA
e-mail: ssimsek@purdue.edu

S. C. Pak et al. (eds.), *Modified Rice Bran Arabinoxylan*,
https://doi.org/10.1007/978-981-19-5735-2_1

1.1 Rice

Cereal grains comprise over 73% of the total world agricultural crops, and they provide dietary fiber, energy, proteins, and other bioactive components required for human health (Charalampopoulos et al. 2002). Rice (*Oryza sativa* L.) is a major cereal, and it is a staple food for more than half of the world's population (Wani et al. 2012). It has been reported that more than 2 billion people obtain 75% of their daily calorie intake from rice in Asian countries (Roy et al. 2011). As a result, rice is grown in more than 100 countries and is used mainly for human dietary consumption (Chang 2002). Rice contains 80% carbohydrates, 7–8% proteins, 3% fat, and 3% fiber (Juliano and Bechtel 1985), and rice grain contains about 5% bran, of which 12–18.5% is oil (Saikia and Deka 2011). The milling of rice yields low-value byproducts/wastes, such as bran and seed coat. Rice bran is a mixture of bran and germ that remains after the removal of husk and the endosperm during milling (Mccaskill and Zhang 1999).

1.2 Rice Bran

Rice bran is a good source of proteins, minerals, fatty acids, and dietary fiber (Mccaskill and Zhang 1999). Rice bran represents 5–8% of the total grain. It is primarily composed of aleurone, pericarp, sub-aleurone layer, and germ (Gul et al. 2016). It was estimated that global rice production is 741 million tons, with more than 70 million tons of rice bran extracted in 2014 (Food and Agriculture Organization (FAO) 2015). However, some studies stated that rice bran has a global potential to produce about 29.3 million tons annually. Rice bran is attracting attention in research due to several reasons including its excellent nutrient composition, easy availability, low cost, high antioxidant potential, and health beneficial effects (Sohail et al. 2017). Approximate composition analysis of rice bran and its derivatives shows that oils (20–29%), carbohydrates (20–27%), and proteins (10–15%) are the three major components (Taha et al. 2012). Moreover, rice bran is also rich in B-complex vitamins (Saunders 1985). The rice bran contains minerals including iron, phosphorus, and magnesium and approximately 11.5% fibers (Oliveira et al. 2011). The composition of rice bran depends upon several factors including rice type, climatic conditions, and rice processing methods (Grist 1985).

Rice bran is an excellent nutrient source, but it is not suitable for human consumption due to the rancidity caused by the presence of lipase enzymes. During milling, bran layers are removed from the endosperm; as a result, the individual cells are disrupted, and lipase enzymes come into contact with fat and initiate the hydrolysis of fat to free fatty acids and glycerol (Malekian et al. 2000). In addition, rice bran does not masticate well because of possible hull contamination. Therefore, it has been estimated that 90% of the rice bran produced in the world is utilized cheaply as a feedstock for cattle and poultry, and the remainder is used for extraction of rice bran oil (Schramm et al. 2007; Zullaikah et al. 2009).

Rice bran hemicelluloses and preparations from defatted rice bran have a great potential in the food industry due to the presence of fibers, especially in the development of functional foods such as functional bakery products (Hu et al. 2009). It can be used in the production of low-fat and high-fiber bakery products (Keneddy et al. 1996). Moreover, industrially, it is used in meat emulsions and batter mixes (Tuncel et al. 2014). Rice bran affects the functional properties of foods such as texture, gelling, thickening, emulsifying, and stabilizing qualities of certain foods (Dreher 1987; Sharma 1981).

Fermented rice bran is used as a new food adjunct as it contains many essential amino acids for humans (Kim et al. 2001). Different food products could be produced to contain 5–10% rice bran (Lebesi and Tzia 2011; Gordon 1989; Hallén et al. 2004; International Organization for Standardization (ISO) 1998). It is considered as an underutilized source of dietary fiber compared to other cereal brans such as wheat, rye, and corn. Therefore, it is appealing to enrich foods with dietary fiber from rice bran as a food ingredient due to its functional and nutritional potential and being a less expensive source of dietary fiber than other cereal brans (Chinma et al. 2015).

1.3 Rice Bran Dietary Fiber

Dietary fiber are nondigestible polysaccharides which are indigestible by human gut enzymes. In cereals, non-starch polysaccharides make up to 75% of the cell wall and is mainly composed of glucomannan, (1–3)- and (1–4)-linked β glucan, cellulose, and arabinoxylans (Pedersen et al. 2014). Rice bran dietary fiber is mainly composed of cellulose, hemicellulose, lignin, and pectin (Chinma et al. 2015; Elleuch et al. 2011). The total dietary fiber content in stabilized rice bran ranges from 25 to 40% depending on the product (Carroll 1990). Most of the dietary fiber of rice bran is insoluble, and soluble fiber comprises only about 7–13% (Anderson et al. 1990). The recommendation for total dietary fiber intake is 38 g/d and 25 g/d for young men and women, respectively (Slavin 2005).

It has been reported that increased intake of dietary fiber has beneficial effects against several chronic diseases. Higher dietary fiber intake lowers blood pressure and serum cholesterol levels and improves glycemia and insulin sensitivity in nondiabetic and diabetic individuals. Furthermore, increasing consumption of dietary fiber has significant benefits on gastroesophageal reflux disease, duodenal ulcer, diverticulitis, constipation, and hemorrhoids and enhances immune function (Anderson et al. 2009). Furthermore, dietary fiber has been accepted in the prevention and management of noncommunicable diseases in Western society as dietary fiber exerts its direct physiological effect throughout the gastrointestinal tract in addition to affecting metabolic activities. These mechanisms of action are related to its physicochemical properties and its fermentation in the large intestine (Guillon and Champ 2000).

1.4 Rice Bran Arabinoxylans

Arabinoxylan content in rice bran is about 4.84–8.5% (Hashimoto et al. 1987), whereas it has been also reported to be as high as 10% in some studies (Malathi and Devegowda 2001; Mansberger et al. 2014). Arabinoxylans are the major non-starch polysaccharides found in cereals and are composed of backbone chains of β-(1–4)-linked D-xylopyranosyl residues that can be substituted with α-L-arabino furanose units through α-(1,2) and/or α-(1,3) glycosidic linkages as side chains in the second and/or third carbon positions (Courtin et al. 2000; Roubroeks et al. 2000; Zhou et al. 2010). Therefore, there are both mono- and di-substituted xylopyranosyl residues at the O-2 and O-3 positions and non-substituted xylopyranosyl residues. The majority of L-arabino furanose substitutions are monomeric, whereas a small proportion of substitutions can form short oligomers, which consist of two or more arabino furanose residues or an arabino furanose residue with a terminal xylopyranosyl residue (Broekaert et al. 2011; Saulnier et al. 2007). In contrast, other rare substitutions include the linkage of glucuronic acids, uronic acids, D-galactose, D-glucose, and acetyl residues to the xylopyranosyl backbone at the O-2 and/or O-3 position (Pastell et al. 2009).

Arabinoxylans are classified as either water-extractable arabinoxylans or water-unextractable arabinoxylans depending on their solubility. The structure of water-unextractable arabinoxylans is different from water-extractable arabinoxylans; however, water-unextractable arabinoxylans are solubilized in alkaline solutions (Moza and Gujral 2017). Arabinoxylan contents of different types of rice grain tissues and grain are shown in Table 1.1.

It has been reported that rice bran contains 303 mg/100 g of ferulic acid (Jung et al. 2007) which might affect arabinoxylans' solubility. Recent reports have shown that ferulic acid side chains are esterified to some arabinose residues (Snelders et al. 2013). The solubility of arabinoxylans could also be affected by close packing of the cell content, which is proposed to be due to steric hindrance (Faulds et al. 2006). In contrast, several studies have reported that arabinoxylan's solubility depends on its degree of branching (Mandalari et al. 2005). Arabinoxylans with high arabinose substitution have a higher solubility in water and vice versa. Degree of branching

Table 1.1 Total AX, WEAX, and WUAX contents of rice grain and its byproducts (%)

Tissue/raw material	Total AX	WEAX	WUAX	References
Bran	4.84–5.11 8.5	0.35–0.77 0.2	4.34–4.49 8.3	Hashimoto et al. (1987) Choct (2015)
Defatted pericarp	26.7	NA	NA	Wang et al. (2016)
Defatted aleurone	13.2	NA	NA	Wang et al. (2016)
Hulls	8.36–9.24	0.11	8.25–9.13	Hashimoto et al. (1987)
Cooked	0.5	NA	NA	Dodevska et al. (2013)
Germinated whole grain	2.97–6.84	NA	NA	Kim et al. (2015)
Whole grain	2.64	0.06	2.58	Hashimoto et al. (1987)

NA not available, *AX* arabinoxylans, *WEAX* water-extractable arabinoxylans, *WUAX* water-unextractable arabinoxylans, % dry weight basis and molecular weight distribution of arabinoxylans determine the health benefits such as immunological activities to a large extent (Li et al. 2013, 2015; Ma et al. 2017). The enzymatically modified low molecular weight arabinoxylans extracted from rice bran have desirable health effects. MGN-3/Biobran is an arabinoxylan derived from rice bran with modification by hydrolyzing enzymes from the shiitake mushroom (*Lentinus edodes* mycelia extract) (Ooi et al. 2018).

1.5 Rice Bran Arabinoxylan Compound/MGN-3/Biobran

Production of MGN-3/Biobran includes several steps such as extraction of polysaccharides from defatted rice bran hemicellulose, partial hydrolysis of polysaccharides by the carbohydrate-hydrolyzing enzymes obtained from shiitake mushrooms, and treating with high heat and pressure. MGN-3/Biobran is the most widely studied rice bran polysaccharide. The chemical structure of MGN-3 is shown in Fig. 1.1.

MGN-3 is a natural blend of hemicelluloses, and its structure is composed of a xylose backbone attached to arabinose in its side chain. The molecular weight of rice bran arabinoxylan compound is about 30–50 kDa (Ghoneum and Matsuura 2004; Pérez-Martínez et al. 2015). The biological activities of rice bran arabinoxylans are dependent on their sugar composition, molecular weight, and degree of branching (Zhou et al. 2010; Mendis et al. 2017). The MGN-3 has a low molecular weight with a low arabinose-to-xylose ratio of 0.5 (Zhang et al. 2015).

MGN-3 is developed and manufactured in Japan by Daiwa Pharmaceutical Co., Ltd., and marketed worldwide as a nontoxic food supplement under different brand names such as BioBran (globally), Lentin Plus (Japan/Asia), Ribraxx (Australia/New Zealand), BRM4 (United States), and others (Biobran.org 2020).

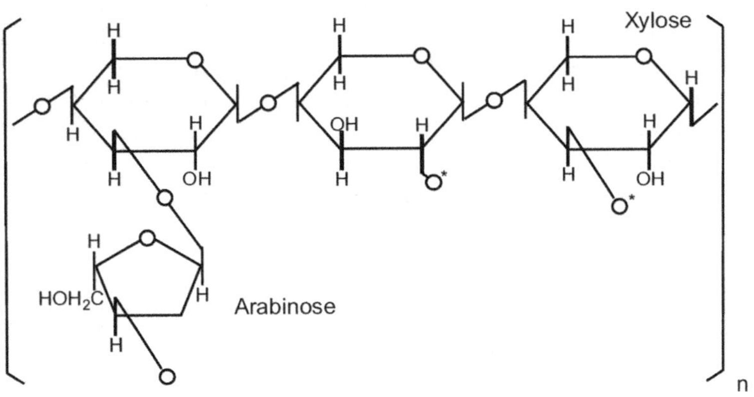

Fig. 1.1 Chemical structure of MGN-3/Biobran (Ghoneum 2014). (Reprinted from Wheat and Rice in Disease Prevention and Health, 1st ed., M. H. Ghoneum, Chapter 31 - Apoptosis and Arabinoxylan Rice Bran, pp 401-408, Copyright 2014, with permission from Elsevier)

The MGN-3 has been identified as a nontoxic compound, and in vivo studies of pig and rat models suggested MGN-3 is negative for mutagenicity, genotoxicity, antigenicity, and subchronic toxicity (Ghoneum 2016). It has been found that >36 g/kg is the lethal dose 50% (LD50) for MGN-3 (BioBran Research Foundation 2013; Daiwa Pharmaceutical Co. Ltd 2020). The safety of MGN-3 was confirmed upon human investigation in clinical trials on cancer patients and analysis of blood chemistry (Ghoneum and Matsuura 2004).

MGN-3 is known to have several health benefits such as anticancer, antiviral, antiproliferative, immunomodulatory, and antioxidant properties. It appears more effective in activating macrophages due to differences in the sugar composition since MGN-3 has more glucose (6%) and galactose (5–7%) side chains compared to other cereal arabinoxylans (Zhang et al. 2015). MGN-3 can activate and enhance host immune system functions by augmentation of macrophage, natural killer cells, T and B cell function, interferon-gamma (IFN-γ), and tumor necrosis factor-alpha (TNF-α) production (Gollapudi and Ghoneum 2008). The anticancer properties of MGN-3 include in vivo cancer cell apoptosis stimulation, tumor growth inhibition in mice, and human breast cancer sensitization to chemotherapy agents. MGN-3 can also enhance antioxidant scavenging enzyme activity along with free radical reduction in tumor-bearing mice with antioxidant disturbances (Ghoneum et al. 2014). MGN-3/Biobran exerts an antioxidant activity against lipid peroxidation, activating the antioxidant defense system and protecting against oxidative stress. MGN-3/Biobran could be used as an antiviral agent as it possesses anti-HIV activity and can inhibit HIV-1 replication by inhibition of HIV-1 p24 antigen production in vitro (Ghoneum 2014).

1.6 Conclusion

Rice bran is one of the most abundant byproducts generated during rice milling process, and it is gaining interest in recent years due to its potential health benefits. Rice bran arabinoxylan compound is a modified form of arabinoxylan and composed of a xylose backbone attached to arabinose monomers with a molecular weight range of 30–50 kDa. The functional and biological activities of rice bran arabinoxylans are highly dependent upon the degree of branching, arabinose-to-xylose ratio, and the molecular weight of the compound. Future studies should focus on studying the fine molecular structure of rice bran arabinoxylans from different rice varieties and using different enzymes. MGN-3 is a modified form of arabinoxylan from rice bran, and there is limited research on the non-modified rice bran arabinoxylans. The modification can be used effectively to improve the activities of MGN-3, providing a new and promising application for rice bran. Moreover, further studies should be carried out to evaluate the relationship between its structure and function.

References

Anderson JW, Deakins DA, Floore TL, Smith BM, Whitis SE (1990) Dietary fiber and coronary heart disease. Crit Rev Food Sci Nutr 29:95–147

Anderson JW, Baird P, Davis RHJ, Ferreri S, Knudtson M, Koraym A et al (2009) Health benefits of dietary fiber. Nutr Rev 67:188–205

BioBran Research Foundation (2013) The safety of Biobran/MGN-3. BioBran/MGN-3 (Rice Bran Arab Coumpound) Basic Clin Appl to Integr Med, 2nd edn. BioBran Research Foundation, Tokyo, pp 9–13

Biobran.org (2020) Biobran MGN-3 - an overview [Internet]. [cited 2020 Oct 18]. https://www.biobran.org/overview

Broekaert WF, Courtin CM, Verbeke K, Van de Wiele T, Verstraete W, Delcour JA (2011) Prebiotic and other health-related effects of cereal-derived arabinoxylans, arabinoxylan-oligosaccharides, and xylooligosaccharides. Crit Rev Food Sci Nutr 51:178–194

Carroll LE (1990) Functional properties and applications of stabilized rice bran in bakery products. Food Technol 44:74–76

Chang T-T (2002) Origin, domestication, and diversification. In: Smith CW, Dilday RH (eds) Rice: origin, history, technology, and production. Wiley, Hoboken, NJ, pp 3–26

Charalampopoulos D, Wang R, Pandiella SS, Webb C (2002) Application of cereals and cereal components in functional foods: a review. Int J Food Microbiol 79:131–141

Chinma CE, Ramakrishnan Y, Ilowefah M, Hanis-Syazwani M, Muhammad K (2015) Properties of cereal brans: a review. Cereal Chem 92:1–7

Choct M (2015) Feed non-starch polysaccharides for monogastric animals: classification and function. Anim Prod Sci 55:1360–1366

Courtin CM, Van den Broeck H, Delcour JA (2000) Determination of reducing end sugar residues in oligo- and polysaccharides by gas–liquid chromatography. J Chromatogr A 866:97–104

Daiwa Pharmaceutical Co. Ltd (2020) Biobran [Internet]. [cited 2020 Oct 18]. https://www.daiwa-pharm.com/english/product/biobran.html

Dodevska MS, Djordjevic BI, Sobajic SS, Miletic ID, Djordjevic PB, Dimitrijevic-Sreckovic VS (2013) Characterisation of dietary fibre components in cereals and legumes used in Serbian diet. Food Chem 141:1624–1629

Dreher ML (1987) Handbook of dietary fiber: an applied approach. Marcel Dekker, New York, NY

Elleuch M, Bedigian D, Roiseux O, Besbes S, Blecker C, Attia H (2011) Dietary fibre and fibre-rich by-products of food processing: characterisation, technological functionality and commercial applications: a review. Food Chem 124:411–421

Faulds CB, Mandalari G, Lo Curto RB, Bisignano G, Waldron KW (2006) Influence of the arabinoxylan composition on the susceptibility of mono- and dimeric ferulic acid release by Humicola insolens feruloyl esterases. J Sci Food Agric 86:1623–1630

Food and Agriculture Organization (FAO) (2015) FAO Rice market monitor. FAO, Rome

Ghoneum M (2014) Apoptosis and arabinoxylan rice bran. In: Watson RR, Preedy VR, Zibadi S (eds) Wheat and rice in disease prevention and health. Elsevier, San Diego, pp 399–404

Ghoneum M (2016) From bench to bedside: the growing use of arabinoxylan rice bran (MGN-3/Biobran) in cancer immunotherapy. Austin Immunol 1:1006

Ghoneum M, Matsuura M (2004) Augmentation of macrophage phagocytosis by modified arabinoxylan rice bran (MGN-3/Biobran). Int J Immunopathol Pharmacol 17:283–292

Ghoneum M, Badr El-Din NK, Ali DA, El-Dein MA (2014) Modified arabinoxylan from rice bran, MGN-3/Biobran, sensitizes metastatic breast cancer cells to paclitaxel in vitro. Anticancer Res 34:81–87

Gollapudi S, Ghoneum M (2008) MGN-3/Biobran, modified arabinoxylan from rice bran, sensitizes human breast cancer cells to chemotherapeutic agent, daunorubicin. Cancer Detect Prev 32:1–6

Gordon DT (1989) Functional properties vs. physiological action of total dietary fiber. Cereal Foods World 34:517–525

Grist DH (1985) Rice, 5th edn. Longman, London
Guillon F, Champ M (2000) Structural and physical properties of dietary fibres, and consequences of processing on human physiology. Food Res Int 33:233–245
Gul K, Singh AK, Jabeen R (2016) Nutraceuticals and functional foods: the foods for the future world. Crit Rev Food Sci Nutr 56:2617–2627
Hallén E, İbanoğlu Ş, Ainsworth P (2004) Effect of fermented/germinated cowpea flour addition on the rheological and baking properties of wheat flour. J Food Eng 63:177–184
Hashimoto S, Shogren MD, Bolte LC, Pomeranz Y (1987) Cereal pentosans: their estimation and significance. 3. Pentosans in abraded grains and milling by-products. Cereal Chem 64:39–41
Hu G, Huang S, Cao S, Ma Z (2009) Effect of enrichment with hemicellulose from rice bran on chemical and functional properties of bread. Food Chem 115:839–842
International Organization for Standardization (ISO) (1998) ISO 13299:1998 sensory analysis — methodology — general guidance for establishing a sensory profile. Geneva
Juliano BO, Bechtel D (1985) The rice grain and its gross composition. In: Juliano BO (ed) Rice chemistry and technology, 2nd edn. American Association of Cereal Chemists, St. Paul, MN, pp 17–57
Jung EH, Kim SR, Hwang IK, Ha TY (2007) Hypoglycemic effects of a phenolic acid fraction of rice bran and ferulic acid in C57BL/KsJ-db/db mice. J Agric Food Chem 55:9800–9804
Keneddy LL, Chung H, Hegsted M (1996) New food product developed from rice bran fractions. IFT Annu Meet B Abstr Abstr Pap Present New Orleans, Louisiana, USA June 22-26, 1996. Institute of Food Technologists, New Orleans, LA, p 56
Kim KM, Yu KW, Kang DH, Koh JH, Hong BS, Suh HJ (2001) Anti-stress and anti-fatigue effects of fermented rice bran. Biosci Biotechnol Biochem 65:2294–2296
Kim MY, Lee SH, Jang GY, Park HJ, Li M, Kim S et al (2015) Effects of high hydrostatic pressure treatment on the enhancement of functional components of germinated rough rice (Oryza sativa L.). Food Chem 166:86–92
Lebesi DM, Tzia C (2011) Effect of the addition of different dietary fiber and edible cereal bran sources on the baking and sensory characteristics of cupcakes. Food Bioprocess Technol 4:710–722
Li W, Hu H, Wang Q, Brennan CS (2013) Molecular features of wheat endosperm arabinoxylan inclusion in functional bread. Foods 2:225–237
Li W, Zhang S, Smith C (2015) The molecular structure features-immune stimulatory activity of arabinoxylans derived from the pentosan faction of wheat flour. J Cereal Sci 62:81–86
Ma J, Adler L, Srzednicki G, Arcot J (2017) Quantitative determination of non-starch polysaccharides in foods using gas chromatography with flame ionization detection. Food Chem 220:100–107
Malathi V, Devegowda G (2001) In vitro evaluation of nonstarch polysaccharide digestibility of feed ingredients by enzymes. Poult Sci 80:302–305
Malekian F, Rao RM, Prinyawiwatkul W, Marshall WE, Windhauser M, Ahmedna M (2000) Lipase and lipoxygenase activity, functionality, and nutrient losses in rice bran during storage. LSU Agric Exp Stn Reports 293
Mandalari G, Faulds CB, Sancho AI, Saija A, Bisignano G, LoCurto R et al (2005) Fractionation and characterisation of arabinoxylans from brewers' spent grain and wheat bran. J Cereal Sci 42: 205–212
Mansberger A, D'Amico S, Novalin S, Schmidt J, Tömösközi S, Berghofer E et al (2014) Pentosan extraction from rye bran on pilot scale for application in gluten-free products. Food Hydrocoll 35:606–612
Mccaskill D, Zhang F (1999) Use of rice bran oil in foods. Food Technol 53:50–51
Mendis M, Leclerc E, Simsek S (2017) Arabinoxylan hydrolyzates as immunomodulators in Caco-2 and HT-29 colon cancer cell lines. Food Funct 8:220–231
Moza J, Gujral HS (2017) Influence of non-starchy polysaccharides on barley milling behavior and evaluating bioactive composition of milled fractions. Food Chem 218:137–143

Oliveira MDS, Feddern V, Kupski L, Cipolatti EP, Badiale-Furlong E, de Souza-Soares LA (2011) Changes in lipid, fatty acids and phospholipids composition of whole rice bran after solid-state fungal fermentation. Bioresour Technol 102:8335–8338
Ooi SL, McMullen D, Golombick T, Pak SC (2018) Evidence-based review of BioBran/MGN-3 arabinoxylan compound as a complementary therapy for conventional cancer treatment. Integr Cancer Ther 17:165–178
Pastell H, Virkki L, Harju E, Tuomainen P, Tenkanen M (2009) Presence of 1→3-linked 2-O-β-d-xylopyranosyl-α-l-arabinofuranosyl side chains in cereal arabinoxylans. Carbohydr Res 344: 2480–2488
Pedersen MB, Dalsgaard S, Knudsen KEB, Yu S, Lærke HN (2014) Compositional profile and variation of distillers dried grains with solubles from various origins with focus on non-starch polysaccharides. Anim Feed Sci Technol 197:130–141
Pérez-Martínez A, Valentín J, Fernández L, Hernández-Jiménez E, López-Collazo E, Zerbes P et al (2015) Arabinoxylan rice bran (MGN-3/Biobran) enhances natural killer cell-mediated cytotoxicity against neuroblastoma in vitro and in vivo. Cytotherapy 17:601–612
Roubroeks JP, Andersson R, Åman P (2000) Structural features of (1→3),(1→4)-β-d-glucan and arabinoxylan fractions isolated from rye bran. Carbohydr Polym 42:3–11
Roy P, Orikasa T, Okadome H, Nakamura N, Shiina T (2011) Processing conditions, rice properties, health and environment. Int J Environ Res Public Health 8:1957–1976
Saikia D, Deka SC (2011) Cereals: from staple food to nutraceuticals. Int Food Res J 30:21–29
Saulnier L, Sado P-E, Branlard G, Charmet G, Guillon F (2007) Wheat arabinoxylans: exploiting variation in amount and composition to develop enhanced varieties. J Cereal Sci 46:261–281
Saunders RM (1985) Rice bran: composition and potential food uses. Food Rev Int 1:465–495
Schramm R, Abadie A, Hua N, Xu Z, Lima M (2007) Fractionation of the rice bran layer and quantification of vitamin E, oryzanol, protein, and rice bran saccharide. J Biol Eng 1:9
Sharma SC (1981) Gums, and hydrocolloids in oil-water emulsion. Food Technol 35:59–67
Slavin JL (2005) Dietary fiber and body weight. Nutrition 21:411–418
Snelders J, Dornez E, Delcour JA, Courtin CM (2013) Ferulic acid content and appearance determine the antioxidant capacity of arabinoxylanoligosaccharides. J Agric Food Chem 61: 10173–10182
Sohail M, Rakha A, Butt MS, Iqbal MJ, Rashid S (2017) Rice bran nutraceutics: a comprehensive review. Crit Rev Food Sci Nutr 57:3771–3780
Taha FS, Mourad RM, Mohamed SS, Hashem AI (2012) Enzymatic pretreatment of stabilized rice bran with mixed enzymes: evaluation of oil. Am J Food Technol 7:452–469
Tuncel NB, Yılmaz N, Kocabıyık H, Uygur A (2014) The effect of infrared stabilized rice bran substitution on physicochemical and sensory properties of pan breads: part I. J Cereal Sci 59: 155–161
Wang J, Suo G, de Wit M, Boom RM, Schutyser MAI (2016) Dietary fibre enrichment from defatted rice bran by dry fractionation. J Food Eng 186:50–57
Wani AA, Singh P, Shah MA, Schweiggert-Weisz U, Gul K, Wani IA (2012) Rice starch diversity: effects on structural, morphological, thermal, and physicochemical properties—a review. Compr Rev Food Sci Food Saf 11:417–436
Zhang S, Li W, Smith CJ, Musa H (2015) Cereal-derived arabinoxylans as biological response modifiers: extraction, molecular features, and immune-stimulating properties. Crit Rev Food Sci Nutr 55:1035–1052
Zhou S, Liu X, Guo Y, Wang Q, Peng D, Cao L (2010) Comparison of the immunological activities of arabinoxylans from wheat bran with alkali and xylanase-aided extraction. Carbohydr Polym 81:784–789
Zullaikah S, Melwita E, Ju Y-H (2009) Isolation of oryzanol from crude rice bran oil. Bioresour Technol 100:299–302

Part II

Therapeutic Properties

Part II aims at detailing the therapeutic properties of RBAC based on scientific evidence from in vivo, in vitro, and human studies.

Enhancing Natural Killer Cell Activity

2

Mamdooh H. Ghoneum

Abstract

Biobran/MGN-3, a unique natural product extracted from rice bran, can strengthen immune health by enhancing the activity of natural killer (NK) cells. NK cells play a crucial role in the first line of defense against cancer and viral infections, but they are suppressed during aging, and low NK cell activity is linked with cancer. Over the last 25 years, studies have shown that Biobran/MGN-3 can enhance this suppression of NK cell activity and furthermore that it has superior effects in comparison with other biological response modifiers (BRMs). Biobran/MGN-3 has been shown to restore the aging-induced NK cell immune suppression of aged mice to normal levels, and it enhanced NK cell activity in human geriatric subjects participating in a randomized, double-blind, placebo-controlled clinical trial. In addition, Biobran/MGN-3 has been shown to exert significant anticancer effects in several studies of mice and rats bearing tumor as well as in human clinical trials against several types of malignancies by a mechanism that involved enhancement of NK cell activity. The molecular mechanisms underlying Biobran/MGN-3's effect on NK cell activity involve increasing the granular content of NK cells and increasing the expression of key cell surface receptors such as adhesion molecule ICAM-1 and the activation-associated receptors CD25 and CD69. Biobran/MGN-3 has no toxicity or side effects, and unlike many other BRMs, its long-term effects are not limited by hyporesponsiveness. This report describes the superiority of Biobran/MGN-3 as a BRM that enhances NK cell activity, followed by evidence showing how

M. H. Ghoneum (✉)
Department of Surgery, Charles R. Drew University of Medicine and Science, Los Angeles, CA, USA
e-mail: mghoneum@g.ucla.edu

S. C. Pak et al. (eds.), *Modified Rice Bran Arabinoxylan*,
https://doi.org/10.1007/978-981-19-5735-2_2

Biobran/MGN-3 can improve lives by reversing aging-induced and cancer-induced NK cell suppression.

Keywords

Biobran/MGN-3 · Cancer · Aging · Biological response modifier · Immunomodulator · ICAM-1

2.1 Introduction

The field of immunotherapy has undergone several phases of development over the past 50 years. From the mid-1970s to early 1990s, the field developed by studying microbes as adjuvant immunotherapy for the treatment of cancer. Microbes such as *Corynebacterium parvum* and *Mycobacterium bovis* (bacillus Calmette-Guérin) were used to treat melanoma (Fahey et al. 1976; Lipton et al. 1983, 1991). From the early 1980s to 1990s, the immunotherapy of cancer also involved studying interleukin (IL)-2 and lymphokine-activated killer (LAK) cells. Dr. Rosenberg developed LAK cell therapy for the treatment of cancer (Rosenberg 1988). However, this therapy was not widely used because it was associated with extremely toxic side effects that included hypotension and required intensive nursing care in 75% of patients (Margolin et al. 1989). More recently, immune checkpoint inhibitors have been studied in the treatment of different tumor types. Unfortunately, this phase of immunotherapy development has also seen that treatment with immune checkpoint inhibitor drugs, anti-CTLA-4 antibodies, and anti-PD-1/PD-L1 agents is associated with severe immune-related adverse events, including fatalities in some cases (Bertrand et al. 2015; Wang et al. 2017). There is a strong need to find and explore safe and effective substances that modify the immune system or "biological response modifiers" (BRMs). Biobran/MGN-3 may satisfy this need: it is a safe, nontoxic BRM that can enhance natural killer (NK) cell activity for long times.

NK cells play a crucial role in the first line of defense against cancer and viral infections by mediating spontaneous cytotoxicity against a variety of malignant tumors and virally infected cells (Trotta et al. 1998; Dustin and Chan 2000; Finn and Lotze 2001). NK cells are a subset of large granular lymphocytes; they can be easily recognized by their reniform nucleus and the presence of many azurophilic granules in their cytoplasm. NK cells attach to cancer cells, after which they release their granules to form holes that ultimately cause cancer cell death. NK cells express diverse families of antigen receptors, as well as expressing the cluster of differentiation molecule CD16 to allow for binding to antibody-ligated target cells. There are several lines of evidence from the scientific literature showing that low NK cell activity is associated with the development of cancer. As a few examples: (1) mouse models with defects in NK cell effector function clearly demonstrate an increased susceptibility to neoplastic disease as they age (Trapani and Voskoboinik 2007); (2) an 11-year follow-up study of a general population indicated that cancer is more likely to develop if NK cell activity is low (Imai et al. 2000); and (3) NK cell activity in cancer patients is significantly decreased compared with that in healthy individuals (Whiteside and Herberman 1994).

The capability of BRMs to be adoptively transferred and augment NK cell activity in vivo has made them the object of great interest, given their potential therapeutic value in treating tumors and in curing different types of malignancies and viral infections. However, the high toxicity of these agents and their common quality of hyporesponsiveness have limited their usage. In the current review, we present data on the augmentation of NK cell activity by the natural supplement Biobran/MGN-3, a prominent immunomodulator with no side effects nor susceptibility to hyporesponsiveness (Ghoneum 1998a, b). Treatment with Biobran/MGN-3 may provide more effective use of signal transduction to mediate tumor cell destruction. We will discuss two important topics: (1) the superiority of Biobran/MGN-3 in comparison with other BRMs and (2) Biobran/MGN-3's ability to reverse aging- and cancer-induced NK cell suppression. The clinical relevance of low NK cell function is of great concern and suggests that balanced immune function (normal NK cell activity) is ideal for good health.

2.2 Superiority of Biobran/MGN-3 in Comparison with Other BRMs

We conducted a literature search of the immunomodulatory effect of 11 BRMs, specifically with respect to NK cell activity. These 11 BRMs were active hexose correlated compound (AHCC), vitamin C, maleic anhydride divinyl ether (MVE-2), *C. parvum*, *Propionibacterium acnes* (*P. acnes*), polyinosinic:polycytidylic acid stabilized with poly-L-lysine (PolyICLC), mouse alpha beta-interferon (IFN-alpha/beta), recombinant IFN (rIFN), recombinant human IFN (rHu IFN), and recombinant human IL-2 (rHu IL-2). These were then compared against Biobran/MGN-3 with respect to (a) extent of NK cell activation, (b) duration of NK cell activation, and (c) hyporesponsiveness.

(a) *Extent of NK cell activation.* In subjects with hypoactive NK cell activity, Biobran/MGN-3 can restore their NK cell activity to normal levels. The extent of this NK enhancement was much higher as compared to other products such as AHCC (Terakawa et al. 2008).
(b) *Duration of NK cell activation.* Studies investigating the immune modulation of Biobran/MGN-3 versus vitamin C showed that one dose of Biobran/MGN-3 increased NK cell activity for 2 weeks in comparison to vitamin C which only increased activity for 24 h (Vojdani and Ghoneum 1993).
(c) *Hyporesponsiveness.* Hyporesponsiveness is characterized by a diminished degree of responsiveness to a stimulus over time. For example, a single administration of a BRM may significantly enhance NK cell activity in the short term, while repeated administrations of the same BRM over time will only result in depression of NK cell activity over the long term. Many BRMs show hyporesponsiveness, including MVE-2, *C. Parvum*, *P. acnes*, PolyICLC, mouse IFN-alpha/beta, r IFN, rHu IFN, and rHu IL-2 (Brunda and Rosenbaum

1984; Talmadge et al. 1985; Saito et al. 1985a, b). It is of great interest to note that Biobran/MGN-3 does not exert hyporesponsiveness. Repeated administrations of Biobran/MGN-3 do not result in decreased NK cell activity, but rather they help to maintain NK cell activity at a high level. This was confirmed in a follow-up study of eight patients with breast cancer, where the patients were treated with Biobran/MGN-3 for 5 years and maintained an elevated NK cell activity relative to baseline over the entire time frame (Fig. 2.1) (Ghoneum and Brown 1999; Ghoneum 1999).

2.3 Biobran/MGN-3 Reverses Aging- and Cancer-Induced NK Cell Suppression

2.3.1 Aging

The geriatric population faces increased incidence of cancer and infections due to the immune deficiencies that come with aging. This is a multifactorial problem, where the loss of immunological vigor plays an essential role in the abovementioned diseases. Studies have shown a clear association between aging and decreased NK cell activity (Ghoneum et al. 1987, 1989, 1991a, b; Itoh et al. 1982; Albright and Albright 1983; Elsaid et al. 2018).

Biobran/MGN-3 has been shown to augment NK cell activity in aged mice and humans. When treatment with Biobran/MGN-3 was introduced to aged mice, a distinct reversal in NK cell activity was observed in as early as 2 days, with the activity increasing from 5.8 LUs before treatment to 35.2 LUs (Ghoneum and Abedi 2004). Biobran/MGN-3 has also been shown to counteract the decline in NK/NKT cell activity in human geriatric subjects given Biobran/MGN-3 at 500 mg/day for 30 days. Specifically, Biobran/MGN-3 enhanced the cytotoxic activity of induced NK cell expression of CD107a (Elsaid et al. 2018).

Further studies aimed to elucidate the mechanisms by which Biobran/MGN-3 functions on NK cell activation. It has been reported that aging is associated with a decline in the perforin expression in aged human NK cells (Rukavina et al. 1998) and with an impairment in perforin secretion, which has been associated with defective polarization of lytic granules towards the immunological synapse (Hazeldine et al. 2012). Example images of degranulated and regranulated NK cells are shown in Fig. 2.2a, b. Studies have shown that the peritoneal NK cells of Biobran/MGN-3-treated aged mice demonstrate an increase in NK cell granular content, as indicated by a remarkable increase in BLT-esterase activity (Fig. 2.2b) (Ghoneum and Abedi 2004). In addition, the increase in NK cell activity may be attributed to an increase in the expression of adhesion molecule ICAM-1 on NK cells (Ghoneum and Jewett 2000).

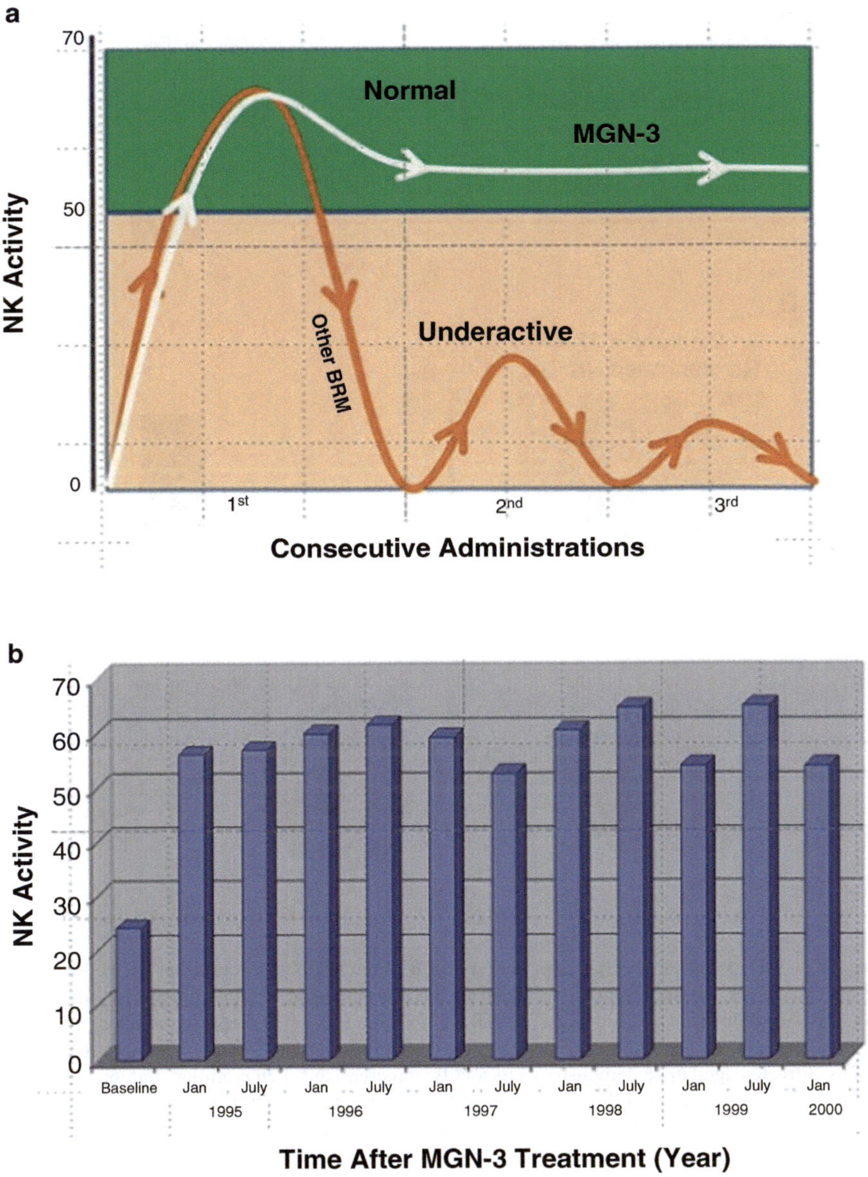

Fig. 2.1 Effect of long-term Biobran/MGN-3 treatment on human NK cell activity. (**a**) Schematic representation of NK cell activity in response to long-term BRM treatment and the general difference between the long-term trends observed with Biobran/MGN-3 versus other BRMs. (**b**) Eight patients with breast cancer were treated with Biobran/MGN-3 at a concentration of 45 mg/kg/day for 5 years. NK cell activity was examined biannually and was measured by standard 51Cr-release assay using K562 cell line as targets. Notice the maintenance of NK cell activity at high levels post-treatment with Biobran/MGN-3 as compared with the baseline value

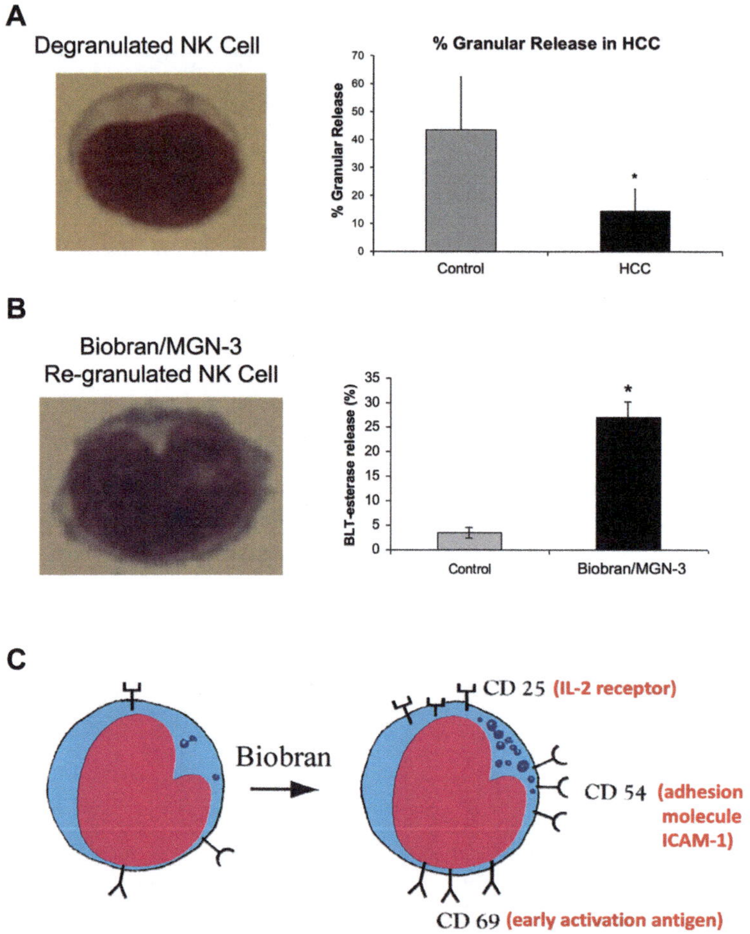

Fig. 2.2 The molecular mechanisms underlying Biobran/MGN-3's action on NK cell activity in aging and cancer. (**a**) Representation of decreased NK granularity; Hepatocellular carcinoma (HCC) significantly reduces granular release by NK cells (*$p < 0.01$). (**b**) Representation of an NK cell regranulated by the action of Biobran/MGN-3; the increase in BLT-esterase activity for Biobran/MGN-3-treated aged mice demonstrates its ability to increase NK cell granular content. (**c**) Biobran/MGN-3 treatment increases the expression of key cell surface receptors on NK cells. Addition of Biobran/MGN-3 to NK cells for 16 h results in increased expression of CD25 (the interleukin-2 receptor), CD54 (the adhesion molecule ICAM-1), and CD69 (an early activation antigen)

2.3.2 Cancer

Cancer consistently ranks among the leading causes of mortality worldwide. The continually high number of annual deaths indicates that conventional cancer therapies are insufficient to completely eradicate the disease. In addition, the most common cancer treatments such as chemotherapy come with a range of toxic side effects. The development of new therapeutics for combating cancer, both with greater efficacy and lower toxicity, is greatly needed.

Our work, along with that of others, has shown that Biobran/MGN-3 exerts significant anticancer effects on animals bearing tumor. For example, Biobran/MGN-3 treatment significantly reduced tumor volumes in mice bearing Ehrlich mammary carcinoma (Badr El-Din et al. 2008), decreased dysplasia and adenocarcinoma in rats with gastric cancer (Badr El-Din et al. 2016), and exerted antitumor effects on animals bearing neuroblastoma in correlation with enhancement of NK cell activity (Pérez-Martínez et al. 2015). More details can be found in the review article (Ghoneum 2016).

Biobran/MGN-3's effectiveness was subsequently studied in several human clinical trials. Supplementation with Biobran/MGN-3 has been shown to enhance NK cell activity in patients with different types of malignancies, including prostate, breast, leukemia, and multiple myeloma (Ghoneum and Brown 1999; Ghoneum 1999; Cholujova et al. 2013). In addition, Biobran/MGN-3 treatment of patients with hepatocellular carcinoma (HCC) showed a significant decrease in tumor volume, decrease in patient cancer recurrence, and improvement of patient survival (Bang et al. 2010).

HCC is currently the third leading cause of cancer mortality, and studies have shown that the abnormal expression of NK cell receptors and dysfunction of liver NK cells are significantly associated with poor prognosis for liver cancer and contribute to the progression of chronic HBV infection and HCC (Ghoneum et al. 1996; Sun et al. 2015). We hypothesize that Biobran/MGN-3 interferes in the signal transduction pathway. Studies have shown that the levels of CD3, IL-2, and IFN-γ mRNA in the spleens of chickens fed with Biobran/MGN-3 were higher than those in the control chickens (Sato et al. 2012). Care was taken to determine that the mechanism was not mediated by lipopolysaccharide contamination of Biobran/MGN-3 (Pérez-Martínez et al. 2015; Sato et al. 2012).

Biobran/MGN-3 also increases the expression of different receptors on NK cells. We have shown that Biobran/MGN-3 treatment of NK cells for 16 hours increases their expression of key cell surface receptors, including CD69 (an early activation antigen), CD25 (the interleukin-2 receptor), and CD54 (the adhesion molecule ICAM-1) (Fig. 2.2c) (Ghoneum and Jewett 2000). Furthermore, NK cells stimulated with Biobran/MGN-3 induced a higher expression of the activation-associated receptors CD25 and CD69 than unstimulated cells. Biobran/MGN-3 promoted NK cell expansion and decreased T cells in vitro, suggesting that Biobran/MGN-3 selectively augments the expansion of NK cells (Pérez-Martínez et al. 2015). These results show that Biobran/MGN-3 (1) increases the granule content of NK cells and (2) increases the expression of cell receptor ligands that can recognize cancer cells, facilitating cancer cell destruction. They also suggest that Biobran/MGN-3 can be used as an adjuvant to existing immunotherapeutic modalities.

2.3.3 Effective Concentration and Biosafety

Biobran/MGN-3 has been shown to enhance NK cell activity at concentrations of 15, 30, and 45 mg/kg (or 1, 2, and 3 gm) per day (Ghoneum 1998b). However, later studies have also shown that Biobran/MGN-3 is even effective at low concentrations of 500 mg/day for significantly enhancing NK cell activity (Elsaid et al. 2018).

Biobran/MGN-3 has been shown to be a safe and nontoxic agent as manifested by the following: (1) the LD50 (lethal dose, 50%) of Biobran/MGN-3 is greater than 36 g/kg; (2) the Ames test for mutagenicity was negative; and (3) the subchronic toxicity study (28-day dietary study in beagle dogs), the guinea pig antigenicity study, and genotoxic testing all demonstrate that Biobran/MGN-3 is nontoxic (Daiwa Pharmaceutical Co. Ltd 2020; Tazawa 2006). Furthermore, Biobran/MGN-3 was examined for toxicity in humans using blood chemistry analysis utilizing Panel 20, which includes liver enzymes (SGOT and SGPT). After 1 month of treatment, no abnormalities were detected for these parameters in comparison to baseline (Ghoneum 1998b).

Earlier studies have also shown the potential for Biobran/MGN-3 in reducing chemo-toxic effects in murine and cancer patients, including protection against severe weight loss induced by cisplatin and adriamycin in animals (Jacoby et al. 2001; Endo and Kanbayashi 2003). In addition, cancer patients treated with chemotherapy and Biobran/MGN-3 have shown marked improvement in appetite and other quality of life parameters (Takahara and Sano 2004; Hajtó et al. 2016). Biobran/MGN-3 has not shown any adverse side effects after long periods of treatment in animals for 8 months (Badr El-Din et al. 2016) and in humans for 5 years (Ghoneum and Brown 1999; Ghoneum 1999).

In 1991, the National Cancer Institute and the National Institutes of Health called for grant applications to study anticancer model development, stating that "Cancer treatments with greater specificity for cancer cells and less toxicity for normal tissues are critically needed" (National Cancer Institute 1991). This statement is as true 30 years later as it was in 1991. We believe that Biobran/MGN-3 in conjunction with other modalities offers great beneficial effects for cancer immunotherapy and is a step towards this critical need.

2.4 Conclusion

Biobran/MGN-3, a novel BRM from rice bran, reverses aging- and cancer-induced NK cell suppression. Supplementation with Biobran/MGN-3 is therefore an effective tool to help combat the immunological effects of aging and cancer through NK cell immunomodulation. The evidence from many studies strongly suggests that this natural, safe, nontoxic product would be useful for future NK cell therapeutic strategies for treating cancer and that Biobran/MGN-3 should be used as an adjuvant to existing immunotherapeutic modalities for cancer patients.

References

Albright JW, Albright JF (1983) Age-associated impairment of murine natural killer activity. Proc Natl Acad Sci U S A 80:6371–6375

Badr El-Din NK, Noaman E, Ghoneum M (2008) In vivo tumor inhibitory effects of nutritional rice bran supplement MGN-3/Biobran on ehrlich carcinoma-bearing mice. Nutr Cancer 60:235–244

Badr El-Din NK, Abdel Fattah SM, Pan D, Tolentino L, Ghoneum M (2016) Chemopreventive activity of MGN-3/Biobran against chemical induction of glandular stomach carcinogenesis in rats and its apoptotic effect in gastric cancer cells. Integr Cancer Ther 15:NP26. https://doi.org/10.1177/1534735416642287

Bang MH, Van RT, Thinh NT et al (2010) Arabinoxylan rice bran (MGN-3) enhances the effects of interventional therapies for the treatment of hepatocellular carcinoma: a three-year randomized clinical trial. Anticancer Res 30:5145–5151

Bertrand A, Kostine M, Barnetche T, Truchetet M-E, Schaeverbeke T (2015) Immune related adverse events associated with anti-CTLA-4 antibodies: systematic review and meta-analysis. BMC Med 13:211

Brunda MJ, Rosenbaum D (1984) Modulation of murine natural killer cell activity in vitro and in vivo by recombinant human interferons. Cancer Res 44:597–601

Cholujova D, Jakubikova J, Czako B, Martisova M, Hunakova L, Duraj J, Mistrik M, Sedlak J (2013) MGN-3 arabinoxylan rice bran modulates innate immunity in multiple myeloma patients. Cancer Immunol Immunother 62:437–445

Daiwa Pharmaceutical Co. Ltd (2020) Biobran. https://www.daiwa-pharm.com/english/product/biobran.html. Accessed 18 Oct 2020

Dustin ML, Chan AC (2000) Signaling takes shape in the immune system. Cell 103:283–294

Elsaid AF, Shaheen M, Ghoneum M (2018) Biobran/MGN-3, an arabinoxylan rice bran, enhances NK cell activity in geriatric subjects: a randomized, double-blind, placebo-controlled clinical trial. Exp Ther Med 15:2313–2320

Endo Y, Kanbayashi H (2003) Modified rice bran beneficial for weight loss of mice as a major and acute adverse effect of cisplatin. Pharmacol Toxicol 92:300–303

Fahey JL, Brosman S, Ossorio RC, O'Toole C, Zighelboim J (1976) Immunotherapy and human tumor immunology. Ann Intern Med 84:454–465

Finn OJ, Lotze MT (2001) A decade in the life of tumor immunology. Clin Cancer Res 7:759s–760s

Ghoneum M (1998a) Anti-HIV activity in vitro of MGN-3, an activated arabinoxylane from rice bran. Biochem Biophys Res Commun 243:25–29

Ghoneum M (1998b) Enhancement of human natural killer cell activity by modified arabinoxylane from rice bran (MGN-3). Int J Immunother 14:89–99

Ghoneum M (1999) Immunostimulation and cancer prevention. 7th international congress on anti-aging & biomedical technologies, 11–13 December, Las Vegas, NV, USA

Ghoneum M (2016) From bench to bedside: the growing use of arabinoxylan rice bran (MGN-3/Biobran) in cancer immunotherapy. Austin Immunol 1:1006

Ghoneum M, Abedi S (2004) Enhancement of natural killer cell activity of aged mice by modified arabinoxylan rice bran (MGN-3/Biobran). J Pharm Pharmacol 56:1581–1588

Ghoneum M, Brown J (1999) NK Immunorestoration and cancer patients by BioBran/MGN-3, a modified aracbynoxylan rice bran (Study of 32 patients followed for up to 4 years). In: Klatz RM, Goldman R (eds) Anti-aging medical therapeutics, vol III. Health Quest Publications, Marina del Rey, CA, pp 217–226

Ghoneum M, Jewett A (2000) Production of tumor necrosis factor-alpha and interferon-gamma from human peripheral blood lymphocytes by MGN-3, a modified arabinoxylan from rice bran, and its synergy with interleukin-2 in vitro. Cancer Detect Prev 24:314–324

Ghoneum M, Gill G, Wojdani A, Payne C, Alfred LJ (1987) Suppression of basal and corynebacterium parvum-augmented NK activity during chemically induced tumor development. Int J Immunopharmacol 9:71–78

Ghoneum M, Salem F, Gill G, Jackson K, Betru Y, Allen H (1989) NK cell activity and tumor development of age-related variation to 3-methylcholanthrene. In: Ades EW, Lopez C (eds) Natural killer cells and host defense: 5th international natural killer cells workshop, Hilton Head, NC, March 1988. Karger, Basel, pp 278–284

Ghoneum M, Jackson K, Salem F, Gill G (1991a) Murine inter-sex difference in methylcholanthrene induced tumor and its correlation with NK activity. Int J Immunopathol Pharmacol 4:9–18

Ghoneum M, Suzuki K, Gollapudi S (1991b) Phorbol myristate acetate corrects impaired NK function of old mice. Scand J Immunol 34:391–397

Ghoneum M, Ghonaim M, Namatalla G, Vojdani A, Alamy M (1996) NK cell activity in hepatocellular carcinoma and its relation to the etiology of the disease. J Clean Technol Environ Toxicol Occup Med 5:267–284

Hajtó T, Horvath A, Papp S (2016) Improvement of quality of life in tumor patients after an immunomodulatory treatment with standardized mistletoe lectin and arabinoxylan plant extracts. Int J Neurorehabilitation 3:2–4

Hazeldine J, Hampson P, Lord JM (2012) Reduced release and binding of perforin at the immunological synapse underlies the age-related decline in natural killer cell cytotoxicity. Aging Cell 11:751–759

Imai K, Matsuyama S, Miyake S, Suga K, Nakachi K (2000) Natural cytotoxic activity of peripheral-blood lymphocytes and cancer incidence: an 11-year follow-up study of a general population. Lancet 356:1795–1799

Itoh K, Suzuki R, Umezu Y, Hanaumi K, Kumagai K (1982) Studies of murine large granular lymphocytes. II. Tissue, strain, and age distributions of LGL and LAL. J Immunol 129:395–405

Jacoby HI, Wnorowski G, Sakata K, Maeda H (2001) The effect of MGN-3 on cisplatin and doxorubicin induced toxicity in the rat. J Nutraceuticals Funct Med Foods 3:3–12

Lipton A, Harvey HA, Lawrence B et al (1983) Corynebacterium parvum versus BCG adjuvant immunotherapy in human malignant melanoma. Cancer 51:57–60

Lipton A, Harvey HA, Balch CM, Antle CE, Heckard R, Bartolucci AA (1991) Corynebacterium parvum versus bacille Calmette-Guérin adjuvant immunotherapy of stage II malignant melanoma. J Clin Oncol 9:1151–1156

Margolin KA, Rayner AA, Hawkins MJ, Atkins MB, Dutcher JP, Fisher RI, Weiss GR, Doroshow JH, Jaffe HS, Roper M (1989) Interleukin-2 and lymphokine-activated killer cell therapy of solid tumors: analysis of toxicity and management guidelines. J Clin Oncol 7:486–498

National Cancer Institute (1991) Anticancer model development. NIH Guid 20:8

Pérez-Martínez A, Valentín J, Fernández L et al (2015) Arabinoxylan rice bran (MGN-3/biobran) enhances natural killer cell-mediated cytotoxicity against neuroblastoma in vitro and in vivo. Cytotherapy 17:601–612

Rosenberg SA (1988) The development of new immunotherapies for the treatment of cancer using interleukin-2. A review. Ann Surg 208:121–135

Rukavina D, Laskarin G, Rubesa G, Strbo N, Bedenicki I, Manestar D, Glavas M, Christmas SE, Podack ER (1998) Age-related decline of perforin expression in human cytotoxic T lymphocytes and natural killer cells. Blood 92:2410–2420

Saito T, Welker RD, Fukui H, Herberman RB, Chirigos MA (1985a) Development of hyporesponsiveness to augmentation of natural killer cell activity after multiple doses of maleic anhydride divinyl ether: association with decreased numbers of large granular lymphocytes. Cell Immunol 90:577–589

Saito T, Ruffman R, Welker RD, Herberman RB, Chirigos MA (1985b) Development of hyporesponsiveness of natural killer cells to augmentation of activity after multiple treatments with biological response modifiers. Cancer Immunol Immunother 19:130–135

Sato K, Takahashi K, Aoki M, Kamada T, Yagyu S (2012) Dietary supplementation with modified arabinoxylan rice bran (MGN-3) modulates inflammatory responses in broiler chickens. J Poult Sci 49:86–93

Sun C, Sun H, Zhang C, Tian Z (2015) NK cell receptor imbalance and NK cell dysfunction in HBV infection and hepatocellular carcinoma. Cell Mol Immunol 12:292–302

Takahara K, Sano K (2004) Life prolongation and QOL improvement effect of modified arabinoxylan from rice bran (BioBran/MGN-3) for progressive cancer. Clin Pharmacol Ther 14:267–271

Talmadge JE, Herberman RB, Chirigos MA, Maluish AE, Schneider MA, Adams JS, Philips H, Thurman GB, Varesio L, Long C (1985) Hyporesponsiveness to augmentation of murine natural killer cell activity in different anatomical compartments by multiple injections of various immunomodulators including recombinant interferons and interleukin 2. J Immunol 135: 2483–2491

Tazawa K (ed) (2006) BioBran/MGN-3 (Rice bran Arabinoxylan Deritive): basic and clinical application to integrative medicine, 1st edn. Iyakusyuppan, Tokyo

Terakawa N, Matsui Y, Satoi S, Yanagimoto H, Takahashi K, Yamamoto T, Yamao J, Takai S, Kwon A-H, Kamiyama Y (2008) Immunological effect of active hexose correlated compound (AHCC) in healthy volunteers: a double-blind, placebo-controlled trial. Nutr Cancer 60:643–651

Trapani JA, Voskoboinik I (2007) Infective, neoplastic, and homeostatic sequelae of the loss of perforin function in humans. Adv Exp Med Biol 601:235–242

Trotta R, Puorro KA, Paroli M, Azzoni L, Abebe B, Eisenlohr LC, Perussia B (1998) Dependence of both spontaneous and antibody-dependent, granule exocytosis-mediated NK cell cytotoxicity on extracellular signal-regulated kinases. J Immunol 161:6648–6656

Vojdani A, Ghoneum M (1993) In vivo effect of ascorbic acid on enhancement of human natural killer cell activity. Nutr Res 13:753–764

Wang P-F, Chen Y, Song S-Y, Wang T-J, Ji W-J, Li S-W, Liu N, Yan C-X (2017) Immune-related adverse events associated with anti-PD-1/PD-L1 treatment for malignancies: a meta-analysis. Front Pharmacol 8:730

Whiteside TL, Herberman RB (1994) Role of human natural killer cells in health and disease. Clin Diagn Lab Immunol 1:125–133

Immunomodulatory, Antioxidant, Antiangiogenic, and Antiproliferative Effects of Rice Bran Arabinoxylan

3

Soo Liang Ooi, Sok Cheon Pak, and Peter S. Micalos

Abstract

Rice bran arabinoxylan compound (RBAC) is a functional food produced from hydrolysed rice bran denatured with shiitake mushroom enzymes. RBAC demonstrates strong immunomodulatory properties, particularly for enhancing the natural killer cell activity. Additionally, RBAC can augment phagocytic cellular functions by promoting the growth of macrophage and neutrophil antimicrobial/antitumour phenotypes. Research has also shown that RBAC can modulate the production of many cytokines, including tumour necrosis factor-alpha (TNF-α), interferons (IFN-γ and IFN-λ), and interleukins (IL-2 and IL-12) which have antitumour applications. Moreover, RBAC is an inducer for the maturation and activation of dendritic cells (DCs), which plays a crucial role in priming the adaptive immune response against invading pathogens and cell mutations. As DCs are antigen-presenting cells that activate the T lymphocytes, stimulation of DCs by RBAC can induce CD4+ T cell proliferation and inhibit the immunosuppressing Treg cells in patients with underactive immune responses. While not an antioxidant in its own right, RBAC has also been shown to augment the body's natural antioxidant defence mechanisms against free radicals. RBAC also shows antiangiogenesis effects in blocking the vascular endothelial growth factor pathway and thus inhibiting tumour development. Overall, RBAC is a potent antiproliferative food supplement with strong evidence showing that it can arrest tumour proliferation.

S. L. Ooi · S. C. Pak (✉) · P. S. Micalos
School of Dentistry and Medical Sciences, Charles Sturt University, Bathurst, NSW, Australia
e-mail: spak@csu.edu.au

S. C. Pak et al. (eds.), *Modified Rice Bran Arabinoxylan*,
https://doi.org/10.1007/978-981-19-5735-2_3

Keywords

Nutraceuticals · Antitumour · Macrophages · Cytokines · Dendritic cells · T lymphocytes · Oxidative stress · VEGF

3.1 Introduction

Arabinoxylan is a vital component of rice bran dietary fibres that is known to exhibit many health benefits, including modulating immune responses, lowering cholesterol, attenuating type 2 diabetes, and enhancing absorption of certain minerals (Mendis and Simsek 2014). Unmodified arabinoxylan extracted from hydrolysed defatted rice bran also possesses anti-complementary and anti-inflammatory effects in vivo (Wang et al. 2008; Hoshino et al. 2010). However, with a molecular weight ranging between 10 and 10,000 kDa, the cross-links of many side chains in arabinoxylan make it resistant to extraction by water (Mendez-Encinas et al. 2018). Various techniques are used to remove arabinoxylans from the stable networks of cross-links, such as by using enzymes, alkali solutions, or mechanical methods. The resulting modified hemicellulose and arabinoxylans have lower molecular weights, higher solubility, improved digestibility, and enhanced health-promoting properties (Mendez-Encinas et al. 2018).

One approach to denature arabinoxylan from rice bran is by the use of mycelium enzymes. In one study, rice bran was treated with enzymes cultured from nine different fungi types and tested for macrophage stimulating activities (Yu et al. 2004). Treatment with mycelia enzymes from *Lentinus edodes* (shiitake mushroom) exhibited the highest stimulating activity. Hence, this technique is used in rice bran arabinoxylan compound (RBAC) production as a functional food and nutraceutical commercially. The most well-known is the Biobran/MGN-3 developed by Daiwa Pharmaceutical Co., Ltd., in Japan. Research has shown that RBAC possesses immunomodulating, antioxidant, antiangiogenic, and antiproliferative properties, as presented in this chapter.

3.2 Immunomodulation

RBAC has been shown to enhance innate immunity by upregulating the natural killer (NK) cell activity. Much of the research on this aspect is summarised in the previous chapter. Briefly, experiments from various in vitro and in vivo studies demonstrated that NK cells stimulated with RBAC had increased granularity with improved cytotoxic activity against pathogens and malignant cells (Ghoneum 2014). The evidence is further supported with positive results from clinical case reports and human trials (Ooi et al. 2018).

Additional immunomodulating effects of RBAC also include augmenting phagocytic cellular functions; modulating the production of cytokines, including tumour necrosis factor-alpha (TNF-α), interferons (IFN-γ and IFN-λ), and interleukins (IL-2 and IL-12); promoting T and B lymphocyte proliferation; as well as functioning as a natural adjuvant for dendritic cells (DCs) (Ghoneum 2016).

3.2.1 Phagocytic Cellular Functions

Phagocytosis is the complex process of identifying, ingesting, and eliminating pathogens and dead cells in the body (Gordon 2016; Rosales and Uribe-Querol 2017). Cells specialising in the phagocytosis functions of eliminating microorganisms and presenting them to the adaptive immune system are professional phagocytes, including monocytes, macrophages, neutrophils, and DCs, osteoclasts, and eosinophils (Rosales and Uribe-Querol 2017). They are the first line of immune defence against pathogens and tumour cells in nearly all tissues.

Dysfunctional phagocytosis capacity can lead to the uncontrolled growth of cancer. For instance, the tumour-infiltrating macrophages are predominantly the M2 phenotype associated with tissue remodelling and angiogenesis, instead of the M1 phenotype associated with microbial killing (van Dalen et al. 2018). M2 macrophages release cytokines and chemokines that can suppress antitumour immunity, promote tumour progression, and enhance metastasis (Gordon 2016; Yang and Zhang 2017). Similarly, neutrophil classification involves two polarising states: N1 is antitumour and N2, which is pro-tumour (Wu et al. 2019; Wang et al. 2018). By responding to the stimuli such as the granulocyte colony-stimulating factor or transforming growth factor β, neutrophils can transform into the N2 type to induce higher expression of immunosuppression activity in the tumour microenvironment (Wu et al. 2019).

The ability to alter macrophages' phenotype against malignant cells is a novel pathway to enhance the antitumour immune response (Pathria et al. 2019). RBAC was shown to stimulate macrophage activities in three different models: human macrophage cell line, murine macrophage cell line, and murine macrophages. Each model demonstrated an increased percentage of phagocytosis after treatment with RBAC ($p < 0.05$). The treated macrophages also had improved spreading ability and increased cytokine (TNF-α and IL-6) and nitric oxide production (Ghoneum and Matsuura 2004).

Further experiments confirmed that RBAC could upregulate the phagocytic activity against *Escherichia coli*, by human monocytes and neutrophils, in peripheral blood (Ghoneum et al. 2008). Increased oxidative burst and significant induction of cytokines (TNF-α, IL-6, IL-8, and IL-10) were also detected ($p \leq 0.01$). The treatment of bacteria by RBAC without human phagocytes did not affect the bacteria growth. Hence, the results suggest that RBAC is a potent modulator for phagocytic cellular functions but not an antibacterial agent itself (Ghoneum et al. 2008).

3.2.2 Dendritic Cell Maturation

DCs are professional antigen-presenting cells (APCs). Their primary function is to capture and present antigen materials on the cell surface to activate cytotoxic T cell responses. DCs are messengers bridging both innate and adaptive immune systems (Gardner and Ruffell 2016; Mellman 2013). However, proper maturation and differentiation of DCs from monocytes is needed to provide the necessary stimulatory signals for triggering T cell responses. The tumour microenvironment can impair the stimulatory functions of maturing DCs and thus suppress the adaptive immune response (Gardner and Ruffell 2016; Veglia and Gabrilovich 2017).

RBAC has been shown to stimulate the maturation of DCs. In an in vitro study by Cholujova et al. (2009), immature DCs derived from peripheral monocytes were cultured with various cytokine mixes to induce maturation. Adding RBAC induced DC maturation by downregulating the cluster differentiation molecule CD14 and CD1a antigens on the cell surface and by decreasing the endocytic activity of immature DCs. RBAC also increased expression of maturation marker CD83 and the surface density of co-stimulatory molecules CD80 and CD86 (Cholujova et al. 2009).

Similarly, Ghoneum and Agrawal (2011) also reported that human monocyte-derived DCs treated with RBAC showed a significant ($p < 0.05$) dose-dependent increase in the expression of CD83 and CD86 assessed by flow cytometry. The modulatory effects of RBAC on DC maturation were further examined in a placebo randomised controlled trial (RCT) with 48 multiple myeloma patients (Cholujova et al. 2011, 2013). Participants received 2 g/day of RBAC or placebo for 3 months. The RBAC group showed a steady rise in the percentage of circulating myeloid DCs with a significant ($p < 0.05$) increase in the ratio between myeloid DCs and plasmacytoid DCs, when compared to baseline. In contrast, the placebo group experienced no significant changes. Together, these results suggest that RBAC can be a potent inducer of DC maturation and activation.

3.2.3 Cytokine Modulation

Cytokines are major regulators of the innate and adaptive immune systems that can recognise and destroy cancer cells. Many cytokines, including IL-2, IL-12, IL-15, IL-21, granulocyte-macrophage colony-stimulating factor, and IFN-α, have antitumour and immune signalling properties for clinical applications (Waldmann 2018). The United States Food and Drug Administration approves IFN-α and IL-2 as immunotherapy for treating several types of cancers (Berraondo et al. 2019). Hence, there is an increasing interest in finding novel agents which can affect cytokine activity in the tumour microenvironment.

In vitro and in vivo studies suggest that RBAC can modulate the production of many different cytokines. While activating DCs in vitro, RBAC was also shown to increase the production of pro-inflammatory and immunoregulatory cytokines, including IL-1β, IL-6, IL-10, IL-17, TNF-α, IL-12p40, and low levels of IL-12p70 and IL-2, as well as IFN-γ and IL-29 (Ghoneum and Agrawal 2011, 2014). As an in vitro phagocytosis up-regulator of neutrophils and monocytes against *E. coli*, RBAC also significantly induced ($p \leq 0.01$) TNF-α, IL-6, IL-8, and IL-10 along with an increased oxidative burst (Ghoneum et al. 2008).

In a study which treated human peripheral blood lymphocyte, RBAC was shown to increase TNF-α production significantly ($p < 0.001$) by several folds (20- to >100-fold) and IFN-γ (52- to 66-fold), compared to control (Ghoneum and Jewett 2000). In Ehrlich carcinoma-bearing mice injected with RBAC, the levels of TNF-α and IFN-γ increased with an observed decrease in IL-10, an immune-suppressing cytokine ($p < 0.01$) (Badr El-Din et al. 2008).

In an open-label RCT with 20 healthy participants, levels of IFN-γ, TNF-α, IL-1α, IL-1β, IL-8, IL-10, and epidermal growth factor peaked at 30 days after supplementing with RBAC, but only IFN-γ was significantly higher than baseline ($p < 0.017$) (Ali et al. 2012). Cholujova et al. (2013) assessed the plasma concentration of cytokines in multiple myeloma patients supplemented with 2 g/day of RBAC ($n = 30$) or placebo ($n = 10$). The study reported a significant increase ($p < 0.05$) in the levels of pro-inflammatory cytokines (IL-12, IL-17, IFN-γ, and TNF-α) and anti-inflammatory cytokines (IL-4, IL-6, IL-9, IL-10, and IL-13) in the RBAC group after 3 months of treatment, compared to placebo (Cholujova et al. 2013).

3.2.4 T and B Cell Proliferation

T and B cells are lymphocytes involved in the adaptive or antigen-specific immune response. The APCs' presentation of the antigenic epitope triggers CD8+ T lymphocytes to recognise, attack, and destroy invading pathogens directly. As such, CD8+ T lymphocytes are also known as killer T cells or cytotoxic T cells. Another group of T lymphocytes (CD4+ or helper T cells, Th) secrete cytokines to activate B lymphocytes into plasma cells that release specific antibodies against the invading pathogens. Regulatory T cells (CD4 + CD25+, or Treg) suppress the immune response once the pathogens are destroyed, preventing over-activation (Cano and Lopera 2013). Both T and B cells are highly specialised immune defence cells with different subgroups that respond to various pathogens. They can also retain immunological memory to mount an effective response upon re-encountering any previously recognised pathogens. T and B cells work together to recognise, eliminate, and remember foreign proteins or pathogens, forming the body's acquired defensive mechanisms (Chaplin 2010).

Several human studies have investigated the effects of RBAC on the activation of T and B lymphocytes. Ghoneum (1998) studied five healthy volunteers taking 15 mg/kg/day of RBAC for 2 months. Supplementing with RBAC resulted in a significant ($p < 0.001$) proliferation of peripheral mononuclear cells by 137% to 146%, measured through T and B cell mitogen responses. In another study, five cancer patients ingested 3 g/day of RBAC for 1 month. The post-study T and B cell mitogen responses increased by more than 30% significantly over baseline

($p < 0.001$) (Ghoneum and Brown 1999). As DCs are APCs that activate the T lymphocytes, stimulation of DCs by RBAC can also induce CD4+ cell proliferation as shown in a study by Ghoneum and Agrawal (2011). RBAC-stimulated DCs induced significantly higher granzyme B-positive CD8+ cells than unstimulated DCs ($p < 0.005$). The granzyme B-positive CD8+ cells, primed by RBAC-stimulated DCs, also exhibited higher cytolytic activity as compared to unstimulated DC-primed CD8+ cells ($p < 0.005$) (Ghoneum and Agrawal 2014).

Lissoni et al. (2008) studied the effects of RBAC on various subpopulations of T lymphocytes in an observational study. The study included 22 cancer patients, with 16 having untreatable metastatic solid tumours. Participants consumed 2 g/day of RBAC orally for the first month and reduced to 1 g/day in the second month. This study found no change in the mean cell count of lymphocytes, CD3+, CD8+, and NK cells after 2 months. However, it detected an increase in Th, accompanied by a decrease in Treg cells. These changes were not statistically significant. However, the ratio between Th and Treg significantly increased ($p < 0.025$) at the end of the study compared to baseline. Hence, RBAC may enhance immunity by inhibiting the immunosuppressing Treg lymphocytes in patients with underactive immune response.

3.3 Antioxidation

Oxidative stress occurs when there is a physiological imbalance between oxidants (free radicals or reactive species) and antioxidants (Ighodaro and Akinloye 2018). The body has multiple lines of natural antioxidant defence mechanisms against free radicals. Within cells, there are scavenger enzymes, including superoxide dismutase (SOD), catalase (CAT), and glutathione peroxidase (GPx), which break down free radicals generated through cellular respiration into harmless molecules (Ighodaro and Akinloye 2018). Nonenzymatic scavengers such as ascorbic acid, uric acid, glutathione, alpha-tocopherol, and ubiquinol readily donate electrons to oxidants to prevent harmful chain reactions (Birben et al. 2012). Deoxyribonucleic acid (DNA) repairs enzyme systems, and proteolytic enzymes repair the damage caused by free radicals and reconstitute the damaged cell membrane (Ighodaro and Akinloye 2018). If the antioxidant defence is overwhelmed, free radicals will damage essential biomolecules like DNA, protein, and lipids, leading to multiple disease conditions (Birben et al. 2012).

RBAC can augment the antioxidant defence system. Ethanol solutions of RBAC have previously shown high scavenging rates for hypoxanthine-xanthine oxidase-generated superoxide anion radicals, ferrous sulphate-hydrogen peroxide, and ultra-violet light reaction system-generated hydroxyl radicals (Tazawa et al. 2000). In an animal study with Ehrlich carcinoma-bearing mice, Noaman et al. (2008) reported that RBAC efficiently suppressed tumour growth with an associated normalisation of the lipid peroxidation and glutathione contents.

RBAC has also been shown to enhance the endogenous antioxidant enzyme activity of SOD, GPx, CAT, and glutathione S-transferase in the blood, liver, and tumour tissue, as demonstrated in the study by Noaman et al. (2008). Similarly, RBAC upregulated the messenger ribonucleic acid expression of GPx, SOD, and CAT in the liver, demonstrating the protective properties against cellular oxidative stress (Noaman et al. 2008).

Protection against oxidative stress was also shown in another murine study examining gamma radiation effects (Ghoneum et al. 2013). Exposure to ionising radiation is known to induce oxidative stress that can damage cellular macromolecules leading to the demise of haematopoietic tissues (Shao et al. 2014). Mice exposed to gamma radiation showed significant depression in their full blood count, hypocellularity of bone marrow, and a remarkable decrease in splenic weight. In contrast, pre-treatment with RBAC resulted in protection against such irradiation-induced damages (Ghoneum et al. 2013). In another study, mice were exposed to local high-dose abdominal precision radiation. The group which received RBAC treatment showed significantly higher ($p < 0.05$) levels of total antioxidant capacity, GPx, SOD, and CAT indicators, than the control group, in the serum, as well as jejunal and colonic mucosa (Zhao et al. 2020). Hence, RBAC can augment antioxidant defence to counteract the severe adverse effects and toxicity of radiation therapy as confirmed in a double-blind, placebo RCT with head and neck cancer patients ($n = 65$) undergoing radiotherapy by Tan and Flores (2020). Patients receiving RBAC were shown to achieve significantly better clinical outcomes after radiation therapy, compared to the placebo group, with lower rates of mortality ($p = 0.001$), blood transfusions ($p = 0.001$), hospital admissions ($p = 0.001$), and metastasis ($p = 0.029$).

3.4 Anti-angiogenesis

Angiogenesis is the formation of new capillaries from pre-existing blood vessels. It is a crucial physiological process in wound healing, growth, and female reproductive organs (El-Kenawi and El-Remessy 2013). However, it can also be aberrantly activated in many pathological conditions, most notably cancer and chronic inflammatory conditions (Aguilar-Cazares et al. 2019). Vascular endothelial growth factors (VEGFs) play central roles in the regulation of angiogenesis. VEGF-A, the primary factor for angiogenesis, binds to receptors, VEGFR-1 and VEGFR-2, to regulate endothelial cell proliferation, migration, vascular permeability, secretion, and other endothelial functions (Shibuya 2013). Angiogenesis is vital in tumour survival and proliferation. Hence, anti-VEGF-VEGFR molecules are now widely used clinically to treat cancer patients. However, these antiangiogenic drugs can be double-edged swords which may cause side effects such as hypertension, arterial clots, wound healing complications, gastrointestinal perforation, and fistula (Gardner et al. 2017).

Many rice bran constituents, such as γ-oryzanol, tocotrienol, phenolic compounds, cyanidin, and peonidin, possess antiangiogenic properties (Tanaka et al. 2012; Saji et al. 2019; Miyazawa et al. 2008; Kim et al. 2012). Similarly, RBAC can be a natural angiogenesis inhibitor acting through the VEGF pathway. An in vitro study by Zhu et al. (2017) demonstrated that RBAC significantly inhibited VEGF-induced tube formation in human umbilical vein endothelial cells co-cultured with human dermal fibroblasts. Furthermore, RBAC also suppressed the VEGF-induced proliferation and migration of human umbilical vein endothelial cells in a dose-dependent manner (Zhu et al. 2017). The antiangiogenic mechanism of RBAC operates by reducing the VEGF-induced activation of VEGFR-2 and the downstream proteins of Akt, extracellular signal-regulated protein kinase 1/2, and p38 mitogen-activated protein kinase (Zhu et al. 2017). Therefore, RBAC can potentially mediate angiogenesis, implicated in the pathological progression of conditions such as cancer, cardiac and limb ischaemia, diabetic retinopathy, rheumatoid arthritis, and neoplasms (Pang and Poon 2006).

3.5 Antiproliferation

Sustained proliferation is an integral part of cancer development and progression. Cancer arises from mutated cells that can survive pre-programmed cell death, forming premalignant nodules. A benign nodule can adapt and transit to malignancy by invading surrounding tissues through hypoxia and a favourable acidic microenvironment that promotes growth (Feitelson et al. 2015). As discussed previously, most immune cells can polarise towards either inducing or inhibiting cancer growth (Lakshmi Narendra et al. 2013; Noonan et al. 2008). Phenotypic skewing of these cells happens within the tumour microenvironment. Dysfunction in immune cells ultimately leads to reduced immunosurveillance action towards inhibiting cancer growth. Instead, these immune cells promote angiogenesis and proliferation of the tumour (Shalapour and Karin 2015).

With strong immunomodulating properties, RBAC can activate the immune cells towards their tumour inhibitory activities. In this context, RBAC has been shown to have preventive effects against carcinogenic agents in a murine model. Male albino rats exposed to carcinogenic N-nitrosodiethylamine and carbon tetrachloride showed a loss of liver architecture and cell proliferation in addition to neoplastic changes. However, pre-treatment with RBAC (25 mg/kg body weight) before exposure to these carcinogens revealed a significant ($p < 0.001$) reduction in liver tumour volume (Badr El-Din et al. 2016a). The antiproliferative activities of RBAC have also been demonstrated in vitro (Ghoneum and Gollapudi 2003; Ghoneum et al. 2000) and in vivo (Badr El-Din et al. 2008; Noaman et al. 2008; Pérez-Martínez et al. 2015). In one study, squamous cell carcinoma growth was arrested after incubating in RBAC solutions for up to 72 h (Ghoneum et al. 2000). Cell proliferation stopped with an increase in apoptosis through the CD95 death receptor pathway. In another study, an increase of more than 200% in the apoptosis rate of RBAC pre-treated tumour cells (human T cell leukaemic HUT 78) to the agonistic anti-CD95 antibody was observed. The effect was dose-dependent (Ghoneum and Gollapudi 2003).

In an in vivo experiment, female Swiss albino mice bearing solid Ehrlich carcinoma tumours were treated with intraperitoneal injections of RBAC (Badr El-Din et al. 2008; Noaman et al. 2008). Compared with controls, RBAC-treated mice exhibited a significant delay in tumour growth measured by volume (63.27%) and weight (45.2%), without any observed adverse side effects due to the treatment (Noaman et al. 2008). NOD-scidIL-2Rgnull mice inoculated with neuroblastoma cells were treated with intravenous NK cellular therapy using either fresh NK cells or NK cells activated with RBAC overnight. The mice treated with RBAC activated NK cells had upregulated NK cell activation markers, significant neuroblastoma growth inhibition, and higher survival rates than control groups (Pérez-Martínez et al. 2015).

RBAC has also been shown to work synergistically with other natural antiproliferative agents, such as baker's yeast (Ghoneum and Gollapudi 2005) and curcumin (Ghoneum and Gollapudi 2011). Ghoneum and Gollapudi (2005) performed experiments with several human breast cancer cell lines (MCF-7, ZR-75, HCC70) cultured with baker's yeast in the presence or absence of RBAC. Treatment with added RBAC increased the number of apoptotic cells by multiple-fold (2-fold for MCF-7, 2.5-fold for ZR-75, and 1.8-fold for HCC70) after 2 h, compared to baker's yeast alone ($p < 0.001$). Similarly, the synergistic potential of RBAC and curcumin on human multiple myeloma cell line U266 was investigated. Although both curcumin and RBAC induced apoptosis in U266 cells, combining 50 μg/ml of RBAC with curcumin concentrations of 2.5, 5, and 10 μM resulted in 200%, 220%, and 247% increase in cancer cell apoptosis ($p \leq 0.05$), respectively, compared to control cells treated with either agent (Ghoneum and Gollapudi 2011).

RBAC also has synergistic antiproliferative effects with several chemotherapeutic agents. Gollapudi and Ghoneum (2008) evaluated the sensitising activity of RBAC with daunorubicin against human breast cancer cells (MCF-7 and HCC70 cell lines) in vitro. Treatment with selected concentrations of RBAC (100–1000 μg/ml) for 3 days significantly increased the susceptibility of cancer cells to daunorubicin (5.5-fold for MCF-7 and 2.5-fold for HCC70 cells) compared to those treated with daunorubicin alone ($p < 0.01$). In another study, RBAC worked synergistically with paclitaxel by causing DNA damage in cancer cells, enhancing apoptosis, and inhibiting proliferation. Non-metastatic human breast cancer cells (MCF-7) and metastatic murine breast cancer cells (4TI) were cultured with different paclitaxel concentrations in the presence or absence of RBAC. The results showed that RBAC increased the susceptibility of both types of cancer cells to paclitaxel by over 100-fold (Ghoneum et al. 2014).

Experiments in an animal model further confirm the synergy of RBAC and paclitaxel (Badr El-Din et al. 2016b). In female Swiss albino mice inoculated with Ehrlich ascites carcinoma cells, administering RBAC plus a low dose of paclitaxel was shown to suppress tumour growth by 88% in volume, relative to control ($p < 0.01$). In comparison, the suppression of tumour volume with paclitaxel alone was only 59%, and RBAC alone was 77%. Inhibition of tumour growth post-treatment with both agents, compared with either treatment alone, was associated with a decrease in cell proliferation, an increase in DNA damage, and apoptosis of tumour cells (Badr El-Din et al. 2016b).

RBAC has also been shown to arrest tumour proliferation in clinical observations. In a recent case series reported by Pescatore et al. (2022), 14 patients with various metastatic malignancies were recruited to study the effects of RBAC on circulating tumour cells (CTC), a prognostic biomarker for tracking cancer proliferation. The patients took 1 g/day of RBAC for 10–19 weeks. Twelve participants completed the trial, with two died during the study. The mean CTC level of the 12 participants was significantly lower at the end of the study than baseline (2.33 ± 3.5 vs. 8.33 ± 8.89, $p = 0.0047$). Hence, RBAC can be an antiproliferation therapy that slows cancer progression.

3.6 Conclusion

RBAC is a potent immunomodulator. Available research shows that RBAC can enhance NK cell activity, augment phagocytic cellular functions, modulate cytokine production, promote T and B lymphocyte proliferation, and act as a natural adjuvant for DCs. RBAC is an antiproliferative agent which activates the immune cells towards their antitumour phenotypes. It can also complement the antioxidant defence system to reduce oxidative stress which causes cellular damage and ageing. As an inhibitor to angiogenesis, RBAC can mitigate the pathological development of inflammatory conditions. As such, RBAC can be a valuable natural supplement for the prevention and management of cancer and many chronic conditions.

References

Aguilar-Cazares D, Chavez-Dominguez R, Carlos-Reyes A, Lopez-Camarillo C, Hernadez de la Cruz ON, Lopez-Gonzalez JS (2019) Contribution of angiogenesis to inflammation and cancer. Front. Oncologia 9:1399

Ali KH, Melillo AB, Leonard SM, Asthana D, Woolger JM, Wolfson AH et al (2012) An open-label, randomized clinical trial to assess the immunomodulatory activity of a novel oligosaccharide compound in healthy adults. Funct Foods Heal Dis 2:265–279

Badr El-Din NK, Noaman E, Ghoneum M (2008) In vivo tumor inhibitory effects of nutritional rice bran supplement MGN-3/Biobran on ehrlich carcinoma-bearing mice. Nutr Cancer 60:235–244

Badr El-Din NK, Ali DA, Othman R, Ghoneum M (2016a) Abstract 5259: prevention of hepatocarcinogenesis in rats by arabinoxylan rice bran, MGN-3/biobran. Cancer Res 76:5259

Badr El-Din NK, Ali DA, Alaa El-Dein M, Ghoneum M (2016b) Enhancing the apoptotic effect of a low dose of paclitaxel on tumor cells in mice by arabinoxylan rice bran (MGN-3/Biobran). Nutr Cancer 68:1010–1020

Berraondo P, Sanmamed MF, Ochoa MC, Etxeberria I, Aznar MA, Pérez-Gracia JL et al (2019) Cytokines in clinical cancer immunotherapy. Br J Cancer 120:6–15

Birben E, Sahiner UM, Sackesen C, Erzurum S, Kalayci O (2012) Oxidative stress and antioxidant defense. World Allergy Organ J 5:9–19

Cano RLE, Lopera HDE (2013) Introduction to T and B lymphocytes. In: Anaya J-M, Shoenfeld Y, Rojas-Villarraga A, Levy RA, Cervera R (eds) Autoimmunity: from bench to bedside [Internet]. El Rosario University Press, Bogota. https://www.ncbi.nlm.nih.gov/books/NBK459471/

Chaplin DD (2010) Overview of the immune response. J Allergy Clin Immunol 125:S3–S23

Cholujova D, Jakubikova J, Sedlak J (2009) BioBran-augmented maturation of human monocyte-derived dendritic cells. Neoplasma 56:89–95

Cholujova D, Jakubikova J, Sulikova M, Chovancova J, Czako B, Martisova M et al (2011) The effect of MGN-3 arabinoxylan on natural killer and dendritic cells in multiple myeloma patients. Haematologica 96:S117–S118

Cholujova D, Jakubikova J, Czako B, Martisova M, Hunakova L, Duraj J et al (2013) MGN-3 arabinoxylan rice bran modulates innate immunity in multiple myeloma patients. Cancer Immunol Immunother 62:437–445

El-Kenawi AE, El-Remessy AB (2013) Angiogenesis inhibitors in cancer therapy: mechanistic perspective on classification and treatment rationales. Br J Pharmacol 170:712–729

Feitelson MA, Arzumanyan A, Kulathinal RJ, Blain SW, Holcombe RF, Mahajna J et al (2015) Sustained proliferation in cancer: mechanisms and novel therapeutic targets. Semin Cancer Biol 35(Suppl):S25–S54

Gardner A, Ruffell B (2016) Dendritic cells and cancer immunity. Trends Immunol 37:855–865

Gardner V, Madu CO, Lu Y (2017) Anti-VEGF therapy in cancer: a double-edged sword. In: Simionescu D, Simionescu A (eds) Physiologic and pathologic angiogenesis - signaling mechanisms and targeted therapy [Internet]. IntechOpen. https://www.intechopen.com/books/physiologic-and-pathologic-angiogenesis-signaling-mechanisms-and-targeted-therapy/anti-vegf-therapy-in-cancer-a-double-edged-sword

Ghoneum M (1998) Anti-HIV activity in vitro of MGN-3, an activated arabinoxylane from rice bran. Biochem Biophys Res Commun 243:25–29

Ghoneum M (2014) Apoptosis and arabinoxylan rice bran. In: Watson RR, Preedy VR, Zibadi S (eds) Wheat and rice in disease prevention and health. Elsevier, San Diego, CA, pp 399–404

Ghoneum M (2016) From bench to bedside: the growing use of arabinoxylan rice bran (MGN-3/Biobran) in cancer immunotherapy. Austin Immunol 1:1006

Ghoneum M, Agrawal S (2011) Activation of human monocyte-derived dendritic cells in vitro by the biological response modifier arabinoxylan rice bran (MGN-3/Biobran). Int J Immunopathol Pharmacol 24:941–948

Ghoneum M, Agrawal S (2014) MGN-3/Biobran enhances generation of cytotoxic CD8+ T cells via upregulation of DEC-205 expression on dendritic cells. Int J Immunopathol Pharmacol 27: 523–530

Ghoneum M, Brown J (1999) NK Immunorestoration and cancer patients by BioBran/MGN-3, a modified aracbynoxylan rice bran (Study of 32 patients followed for up to 4 years). In: Klatz RM, Goldman R (eds) Anti-aging medical therapeutics, vol III. Health Quest Publications, Marina del Rey, CA, pp 217–226

Ghoneum M, Gollapudi S (2003) Modified arabinoxylan rice bran (MGN-3/Biobran) sensitizes human T cell leukemia cells to death receptor (CD95)-induced apoptosis. Cancer Lett 201:41–49

Ghoneum M, Gollapudi S (2005) Modified arabinoxylan rice bran (MGN-3/Biobran) enhances yeast-induced apoptosis in human breast cancer cells in vitro. Anticancer Res 25:859–870

Ghoneum M, Gollapudi S (2011) Synergistic apoptotic effect of arabinoxylan rice bran (MGN-3/Biobran) and curcumin (turmeric) on human multiple myeloma cell line U266 in vitro. Neoplasma 58:118–123

Ghoneum M, Jewett A (2000) Production of tumor necrosis factor-alpha and interferon-gamma from human peripheral blood lymphocytes by MGN-3, a modified arabinoxylan from rice bran, and its synergy with interleukin-2 in vitro. Cancer Detect Prev 24:314–324

Ghoneum M, Matsuura M (2004) Augmentation of macrophage phagocytosis by modified arabinoxylan rice bran (MGN-3/Biobran). Int J Immunopathol Pharmacol 17:283–292

Ghoneum M, Tachiki K, Ueyama K, Makinodan T, Makhijani N, Yamaguchi D (2000) Abstract: natural biological response modifier (MGN-3) shown to be effective against tumor cell growth. 8th international congress on anti-aging & biomedical technologies [Internet]. http://www.jafra.gr.jp/eng/bio20.pdf

Ghoneum M, Matsuura M, Gollapudi S (2008) Modified arabinoxylan rice bran (Mgn-3/Biobran) enhances intracellular killing of microbes by human phagocytic cells in vitro. Int J Immunopathol Pharmacol 21:87–95

Ghoneum M, Badr El-Din NK, Fattah SMA, Tolentino L (2013) Arabinoxylan rice bran (MGN-3/Biobran) provides protection against whole-body γ-irradiation in mice via restoration of hematopoietic tissues. J Radiat Res 54:419

Ghoneum M, Badr El-Din NK, Ali DA, El-Dein MA (2014) Modified arabinoxylan from rice bran, MGN-3/Biobran, sensitizes metastatic breast cancer cells to paclitaxel in vitro. Anticancer Res 34:81–87

Gollapudi S, Ghoneum M (2008) MGN-3/Biobran, modified arabinoxylan from rice bran, sensitizes human breast cancer cells to chemotherapeutic agent, daunorubicin. Cancer Detect Prev 32:1–6

Gordon S (2016) Phagocytosis: an immunobiologic process. Immunity 44:463–475

Hoshino Y, Hirashima N, Nakanishi M, Furuno T (2010) Inhibition of degranulation and cytokine production in bone marrow-derived mast cells by hydrolyzed rice bran. Inflamm Res 59:615–625

Ighodaro OM, Akinloye OA (2018) First line defence antioxidants-superoxide dismutase (SOD), catalase (CAT) and glutathione peroxidase (GPX): their fundamental role in the entire antioxidant defence grid. Alexandria J Med 54:287–293

Kim SP, Kang MY, Nam SH, Friedman M (2012) Dietary rice bran component γ-oryzanol inhibits tumor growth in tumor-bearing mice. Mol Nutr Food Res 56:935–944

Lakshmi Narendra B, Eshvendar Reddy K, Shantikumar S, Ramakrishna S (2013) Immune system: a double-edged sword in cancer. Inflamm Res 62:823–834

Lissoni P, Messina G, Brivio F, Fumagalli L, Rovelli F, Maruelli L et al (2008) Modulation of the anticancer immunity by natural agents: inhibition of T regulatory lymphocyte generation by arabinoxylan in patients with locally limited or metastatic solid tumors. Cancer Ther 6:1011–1016

Mellman I (2013) Dendritic cells: master regulators of the immune response. Cancer Immunol Res 1:145–149

Mendez-Encinas MA, Carvajal-Millan E, Rascon-Chu A, Astiazaran-Garcia HF, Valencia-Rivera DE (2018) Ferulated Arabinoxylans and their gels: functional properties and potential application as antioxidant and anticancer agent. Oxidative Med Cell Longev 2018:22

Mendis M, Simsek S (2014) Arabinoxylans and human health. Food Hydrocoll 42:239–243

Miyazawa T, Shibata A, Nakagawa K, Tsuzuki T (2008) Anti-angiogenic function of tocotrienol. Asia Pac J Clin Nutr 17(Suppl 1):253–256

Noaman E, Badr El-Din NK, Bibars MA, Abou Mossallam AA, Ghoneum M (2008) Antioxidant potential by arabinoxylan rice bran, MGN-3/biobran, represents a mechanism for its oncostatic effect against murine solid Ehrlich carcinoma. Cancer Lett 268:348–359

Noonan DM, De Lerma Barbaro A, Vannini N, Mortara L, Albini A (2008) Inflammation, inflammatory cells and angiogenesis: decisions and indecisions. Cancer Metastasis Rev 27: 31–40

Ooi SL, McMullen D, Golombick T, Pak SC (2018) Evidence-based review of BioBran/MGN-3 arabinoxylan compound as a complementary therapy for conventional cancer treatment. Integr Cancer Ther 17:165–178

Pang RWC, Poon RTP (2006) Clinical implications of angiogenesis in cancers. Vasc Health Risk Manag 2:97–108

Pathria P, Louis TL, Varner JA (2019) Targeting tumor-associated macrophages in cancer. Trends Immunol 40:310–327

Pérez-Martínez A, Valentín J, Fernández L, Hernández-Jiménez E, López-Collazo E, Zerbes P et al (2015) Arabinoxylan rice bran (MGN-3/Biobran) enhances natural killer cell-mediated cytotoxicity against neuroblastoma in vitro and in vivo. Cytotherapy 17:601–612

Pescatore F, Prestano C, Kichikova M (2022) RBAC and its role with the immune system. Altern Ther Health Med 28:8–10

Rosales C, Uribe-Querol E (2017) Phagocytosis: a fundamental process in immunity. Biomed Res Int 2017:9042851

Saji N, Francis N, Blanchard CL, Schwarz LJ, Santhakumar AB (2019) Rice bran phenolic compounds regulate genes associated with antioxidant and anti-inflammatory activity in human umbilical vein endothelial cells with induced oxidative stress. Int J Mol Sci 20:4715

Shalapour S, Karin M (2015) Immunity, inflammation, and cancer: an eternal fight between good and evil. J Clin Invest 125:3347–3355
Shao L, Luo Y, Zhou D (2014) Hematopoietic stem cell injury induced by ionizing radiation. Antioxid Redox Signal 20:1447–1462
Shibuya M (2013) Vascular endothelial growth factor and its receptor system: physiological functions in angiogenesis and pathological roles in various diseases. J Biochem 153:13–19
Tan DFS, Flores JAS (2020) The immunomodulating effects of arabinoxylan rice bran (Lentin) on hematologic profile, nutritional status and quality of life among head and neck carcinoma patients undergoing radiation therapy: a double blind randomized control trial. Radiol J 12: 11–16
Tanaka J, Nakamura S, Tsuruma K, Shimazawa M, Shimoda H, Hara H (2012) Purple rice (Oryza sativa L.) extract and its constituents inhibit VEGF-induced angiogenesis. Phytother Res 26: 214–222
Tazawa K, Namikawa H, Oida N, Itoh K, Yatsuzuka M, Koike J et al (2000) Scavenging activity of MGN-3 (arabinoxylane from rice bran) with natural killer cell activity on free radicals. Biotherapy 14:493–495
van Dalen FJ, van Stevendaal MHME, Fennemann FL, Verdoes M, Ilina O (2018) Molecular repolarisation of tumour-associated macrophages. Molecules 24:9
Veglia F, Gabrilovich DI (2017) Dendritic cells in cancer: the role revisited. Curr Opin Immunol 45: 43–51
Waldmann TA (2018) Cytokines in cancer immunotherapy. Cold Spring Harb Perspect Biol 10: a028472
Wang L, Zhang H, Zhang X, Chen Z (2008) Purification and identification of a novel heteropolysaccharide RBPS2a with anti-complementary activity from defatted rice bran. Food Chem 110:150–155
Wang X, Qiu L, Li Z, Wang X-Y, Yi H (2018) Understanding the multifaceted role of neutrophils in cancer and autoimmune diseases. Front Immunol 9:2456
Wu L, Saxena S, Awaji M, Singh RK (2019) Tumor-associated neutrophils in cancer: going pro. Cancers (Basel) 11:564
Yang L, Zhang Y (2017) Tumor-associated macrophages: from basic research to clinical application. J Hematol Oncol 10:58
Yu KW, Shin KS, Choi YM, Suh HJ (2004) Macrophage stimulating activity of exo-biopolymer from submerged culture of Lentinus edodes with rice bran. J Microbiol Biotechnol 14:658–664
Zhao Z, Cheng W, Qu W, Wang K (2020) Arabinoxylan rice bran (MGN-3/Biobran) alleviates radiation-induced intestinal barrier dysfunction of mice in a mitochondrion-dependent manner. Biomed Pharmacother 124:109855
Zhu X, Okubo A, Igari N, Ninomiya K, Egashira Y (2017) Modified rice bran hemicellulose inhibits vascular endothelial growth factor-induced angiogenesis in vitro via VEGFR2 and its downstream signaling pathways. Biosci Microbiota Food Health 36:45–53

Anti-inflammatory Agent

4

Jason Ashworth

Abstract

There is accumulating evidence that rice bran extracts have profound effects on mediating inflammation, with the therapeutic potential of rice bran widely explored in several chronic inflammatory conditions including asthma, diabetes, obesity, dermatitis, arthritis, liver injury, neuroinflammation, and cancer. However, rice bran extracts are often poorly characterised, making it difficult to ascertain which constituents of the extract are contributing to the observed anti-inflammatory properties. Despite this drawback, rice bran arabinoxylans (AXs), or AX-derived compounds such as ferulic acid and feruloylated oligosaccharides, have been identified as principal anti-inflammatory agents in rice bran extracts. Moreover, AX-induced patterns of anti-inflammatory effects involving changes in transcription factor regulation, gene transcription, enzyme activity, or inflammatory cytokine/mediator secretion are beginning to emerge in the research literature. Given the body of published research primarily utilises modified rice bran AX, commonly known as Biobran or MGN-3, there is ample scope to explore a wider range of non-modified rice bran AXs as anti-inflammatory agents in future work. Exploiting the emerging anti-inflammatory properties of rice bran AXs to develop potential treatments or prophylactic therapies for inflammatory diseases is an exciting prospect that warrants further investigation.

Keywords

Inflammation · Anti-inflammatory · Arabinoxylan · Rice bran · Biobran · MGN-3

J. Ashworth (✉)
Department of Life Sciences, Manchester Metropolitan University, Manchester, UK
e-mail: J.Ashworth@mmu.ac.uk

S. C. Pak et al. (eds.), *Modified Rice Bran Arabinoxylan*,
https://doi.org/10.1007/978-981-19-5735-2_4

Rice bran is typically considered a waste by-product of rice processing and often discarded or used in animal feeds. However, it is becoming increasingly apparent that rice bran contains numerous potentially useful substances including dietary fibres (Friedman 2013; Sharif et al. 2014; North et al. 2009). Arabinoxylans (AXs) are major dietary fibres found in many cereals such as rice, wheat, and corn that possess multiple immune-mediating activities (Broekaert et al. 2011; Islam et al. 2008; Lee et al. 2021; Zhang et al. 2015). Several extraction processes are available (including water, alkaline, enzymatic, fermentation, mechanical, and extrusion) to yield arabinoxylan (AX) from rice bran (Zhang et al. 2015; Fadel et al. 2018a). It has been reported that low molecular weight (30–50 kDa) AXs have immunostimulatory and anti-inflammatory effects, both in vivo and in vitro (Elsaid et al. 2018; Ghoneum and Matsuura 2004; Zheng et al. 2012a).

With regard to innate immunity, whether low molecular weight AXs act in an immunostimulatory or an anti-inflammatory manner is likely to be dependent on the target cell/tissue type and status. Cells of the adaptive immune system (including B and T cells) are typically stimulated by AXs (Ghoneum 1998; Ghoneum and Gollapudi 2003), as are cells of the innate immune system (e.g., dendritic and natural killer cells) that bridge both innate and adaptive immunity (Cholujova et al. 2013; Ghoneum and Agrawal 2011). In the absence of pre-existing infection or inflammation, AXs tend to stimulate innate inflammatory cell activity (Ghoneum and Matsuura 2004; Ghoneum et al. 2008). However, during persistent infection (e.g., sepsis) or inflammation, evidence suggests AXs and their constituents act in an anti-inflammatory manner, dampening excessive inflammatory cell activity such as cytokine and protease production (Fadel et al. 2018b; Fang et al. 2012; Udani and Hardy 2006). It has been proposed that due to their structural and molecular weight similarity with polysaccharides of microbial origin, such as bacterial lipopolysaccharide (LPS), AXs may bind to and somewhat activate target cell receptors, leading to moderate immune stimulation in the absence of infection or inflammation (Zhang et al. 2015; Fadel et al. 2018b). For example, toll-like receptor-4 (TLR-4) has been identified as a key potential receptor for AXs, since LPS specifically binds to and activates TLR-4 (Mendis et al. 2016). However, in the presence of infection or inflammation, AXs are likely to dampen the overall inflammatory response by effectively competing with bacterial LPS at TLR-4 (Fadel et al. 2018b).

Modified rice bran AX, commonly known as Biobran or MGN-3, is a novel biological response modifier (BRM) obtained from rice bran after enzymatic treatment with an extract from shiitake mushrooms (*Lentis edodes*) (Ghoneum and Agrawal 2011). Modified rice bran AX of low molecular weight (30–100 kDa) can significantly stimulate both the innate and adaptive immune systems (Cholujova et al. 2009; Ghoneum and Abedi 2004). Biobran/MGN-3 has been shown to stimulate the production of interleukin-10 (IL-10), an anti-inflammatory cytokine, by human peripheral blood phagocytes (Ghoneum et al. 2008). In a murine model of LPS-induced sepsis, treatment with BioBran improved survival rate and was associated with a decrease in pro-inflammatory cytokines, including IL-6 (Udani and Hardy 2006). Similar findings have been confirmed with other cereal-derived

AXs, including those from wheat bran that dampened LPS-induced inflammation through decreased production of nitric oxide (NO), tumour necrosis factor-alpha (TNF-α), IL-6, and IL-12 (Kang et al. 2016). Like MGN-3, hydrolysed rice bran (HRB) arabinoxylan is generated from the digestion of defatted water-soluble rice bran with carbohydrate-hydrolysing enzymes from shiitake mushrooms but over an extended period, resulting in lower molecular weight polysaccharides. Pre-treatment of murine bone marrow-derived mast cells with HRB arabinoxylan has been shown to inhibit *mast cell degranulation*, RelA (p65) phosphorylation, and cytokine (TNF-α and IL-4) production (Hoshino et al. 2010). Ji et al. (2020) showed that arabinoxylans extracted from rice bran by microbial fermentation and acid hydrolysis increased cell viability and IL-10 levels following oral administration by mice and in vitro exposure of murine RAW 264.7 macrophages.

Many studies report the beneficial anti-inflammatory effects of rice bran extracts without identifying which constituent(s) of the extract mediate the observed response (Fig. 4.1a). Similarly, the reported anti-inflammatory properties of rice bran AX (Fig. 4.1b) may be attributable (at least in part) to its ferulic acid phenolic component (Fig. 4.1c), which is the major phenolic compound in rice bran (Lee et al. 2021; Jun et al. 2015). Around 70% of phenolics present in rice bran are esterified to arabinoxylan residues of cell walls, and these are released by enzymatic degradation or microbial fermentation (Webber et al. 2014). Feruloylated oligosaccharides can be released either by the enzymatic or mild acid hydrolysis of AXs. Ferulates isolated from rice bran have been shown to protect against inflammatory contact dermatitis in mice (Akihisa et al. 2000). Ferulic acid from rice bran has anti-inflammatory properties in vitro and in vivo via transcription factor (nuclear factor kappa-B [NF-κB]), enzyme (cyclooxygenase-2 [COX-2] and inducible nitric oxide synthase [iNOS]), and pro-inflammatory cytokine (IL-1β, IL-6, and TNF-α) downregulation (Islam et al. 2011). Ferulic acid also inhibits the production of murine chemokine macrophage inflammatory protein-2 (MIP-2) in LPS-stimulated RAW 264.7 macrophages (Sakai et al. 1997). Feruloylated oligosaccharides released from rice bran AXs induced IL-10 whilst suppressing IL-1β, IL-6, TNF-α, prostaglandin E2 (PGE2), and NO production in LPS-stimulated RAW264.7 cells (Fang et al. 2012). Several pro-inflammatory mediators (NO, IL-6, IL-12, and interferon gamma [IFN-γ]) that are induced in RAW264.7 mouse macrophages following stimulation with hydrogen peroxide or bacterial LPS can be dampened by rice bran phenolic extracts containing predominantly ferulic acid (Saji et al. 2020). Furthermore, Saji et al. (2019) showed that these rice bran phenolic extracts mediate the transcription of key inflammatory genes in human umbilical vein endothelial cells under induced oxidative stress, including upregulated endothelial nitric oxide synthase (eNOS) and downregulated intercellular adhesion molecule-1 (ICAM-1), ectonucleoside triphosphate diphosphohydrolase 1 (otherwise called cluster of differentiation 39 [CD39]), and ecto-5′-nucleotidase (CD73) (Saji et al. 2019). ICAM-1 is responsible for promoting the adhesion of circulating leucocytes to endothelial cells and subsequent transmigration to sites of inflammation, whilst CD39/CD73 regulates purinergic mediators such as adenosine triphosphate (ATP) and adenosine diphosphate (ADP) that initiate a series of pro-inflammatory responses. In contrast,

(A) Rice Bran Extracts

Transcription Factor Regulation
IkappaB-alpha degradation (↓)
IkappaB-alpha phosphorylation (↓)

Gene Transcription
Interleukin-1alpha (↓)
Interleukin-1beta (↓)
Interleukin-6 (↓)
Nitric oxide synthase-2 (NOS-2) (↓)
Nuclear factor kappa-B expression (↓)
Peroxisome proliferator-activated receptor-gamma activation (↑)
Tumour necrosis factor-alpha (↓)

Enzymes
Cyclooxygenase-1 (↓)
Cyclooxygenase-2 (↓)
Inducible nitric oxide synthase (↓)
5-Lipooxygenase (↓)
Matrix metalloproteinase-9 (↓)
Prostaglandin E synthase-1 (↓)

Cytokines & Inflammatory Mediators
C-reactive protein (↓)
Interleukin-1beta (↓)
Interleukin-6 (↓)
Interleukin-10 (↑)
Leukotriene B4 (↓)
Tumour necrosis factor-alpha (↓)

(B) Rice Bran Arabinoxylan (AX)

Transcription Factor Regulation
Nuclear factor kappa-B (↓)
RelA (p65) phosphorylation (↓)
IkappaB-alpha degradation (↓)

Gene Transcription
Cluster of differentiation 14 (CD14) (↓)
Nitric oxide synthase-2 (NOS-2) (↓)
Peroxisome proliferator-activated receptor-gamma activation (↑)

Enzymes
Cyclooxygenase-2 (↓)
Inducible nitric oxide synthase (↓)
Myeloperoxidase (↓)

Cytokines & Inflammatory Mediators
C-reactive protein (↓)
Immunoglobulin E (↓)
Intercellular adhesion molecule-1 (↓)
Interferon gamma (↓)
Interleukin-1beta (↓)
Interleukin-4 (↓)
Interleukin-6 (↓)
Interleukin-8 (↓)
Interleukin-10 (↑)
Interleukin-17 (↓)
Interleukin-18 (↓)
Leukotriene B4 (↓)
Nitric oxide (↓)
Rheumatoid factor (↓)
Tumour necrosis factor-alpha (↓)

(C) Rice Bran AX-Derived Ferulates

Transcription Factor Regulation
Nuclear factor kappa-B (↓)
IkappaB-alpha phosphorylation (↓)

Gene Transcription
Intercellular adhesion molecule-1 (↓)
Cluster of differentiation 39 (CD39) (↓)
Cluster of differentiation 73 (CD73) (↓)
Endothelial nitric oxide synthase (↑)
Nitric oxide synthase-2 (NOS-2) (↓)

Enzymes
Cyclooxygenase-2 (↓)
Inducible nitric oxide synthase (↓)

Cytokines & Inflammatory Mediators
Interferon gamma (↓)
Interleukin-1beta (↓)
Interleukin-6 (↓)
Interleukin-10 (↑)
Interleukin-12 (↓)
Macrophage inflammatory protein-2 (↓)
Nitric oxide (↓)
Prostaglandin E_2 (↓)
Tumour necrosis factor-alpha (↓)

Fig. 4.1 Anti-inflammatory properties of rice bran extracts (**a**), rice bran AX (**b**), and AX-derived ferulates (**c**) showing common, overlapping patterns of anti-inflammatory activity on transcription factor regulation, gene transcription, enzyme activity, levels of cytokines, and inflammatory mediators. The symbol (↑) indicates an upregulated response, and the symbol (↓) indicates a downregulated response eNOS generates protective NO in the vasculature, thereby preventing increased reactive oxygen species (ROS) production in endothelial cells. Thus, the work of Saji et al. (2019, 2020) highlights multiple mechanisms of action through which rice bran AX-derived phenolic compounds may dampen inflammation.

Excessive production of pro-inflammatory cytokines and tissue-destructive proteases is associated with many chronic inflammatory conditions, and the therapeutic potential of rice bran to mediate inflammation has been widely explored. Asthma, atopic dermatitis, and rheumatoid arthritis are inflammatory human disorders that appear to be responsive to the anti-inflammatory effects of Biobran/MGN-3 (BioBran Research Foundation 2013). Black rice bran has been shown to significantly dampen gene and protein levels of iNOS, leading to reduced NO levels both in an in vivo murine model of induced asthma and in LPS-activated RAW 264.7 murine macrophages in vitro (Lee et al. 2015). Black rice bran also inhibits NF-κB expression in a murine model of induced asthma (Lee et al. 2005). In a human study of rheumatoid arthritis, some subjects noted a reduction in disease symptoms that were associated with reduced levels of rheumatoid factor and C-reactive protein (CRP) following 6–12 months treatment with 1–3 g Biobran daily (Ichihashi 2004). In human clinical trials, Biobran has been shown to reduce the progression of skin lesions in atopic dermatitis, and this is associated with a reduction in immunoglobulin E (IgE). Ogawa et al. (2005) found a similar effect by corn-derived AXs in a murine model of atopic dermatitis, suggesting the AXs from a variety of cereal grains (not just rice) have this anti-inflammatory property. Rice bran is also effective at reducing inflammation in other types of dermatitis. For example, injection or ingestion of black rice bran in experimental mice reduces the cutaneous inflammation associated with induced allergic contact dermatitis, resulting in reduced tissue oedema and suppression of leukotriene B4 (LTB4), IL-1β, TNF-α, and IL-6 (Choi et al. 2010). In both an in vivo murine model and an in vitro assay of mast cell (RBL-2H3 cell line) allergic responses, fermented rice bran treatment inhibited mast cell degranulation and mRNA levels of IgE-induced pro-inflammatory markers including TNF-α, IFN-γ, IL-4, and IL-6 (Fan et al. 2010).

There is growing evidence that rice bran can dampen liver-associated inflammation. Oral and intraperitoneal administration of Biobran/MGN-3 and particularly the low molecular weight AX fraction of MGN-3 provided protection of liver injury, and this was associated with reduced hepatic IL-18 gene expression and serum IL-18 levels in male Wistar rats (Zheng et al. 2012b). The low molecular weight AX fraction of MGN-3 inhibited CD14 messenger ribonucleic acid (mRNA) expression, IkappaB-alpha (IκB-α) degradation, NF-κB activation, and c-Jun N-terminal kinase (JNK)/mitogen-activated protein kinase (MAPK) expression in a Wistar rat model of hepatitis (Zheng et al. 2012a). Similarly, ferulic acid protects against induced liver injury in mice (Kim et al. 2011), and subsequent investigations showed dietary supplementation with rice bran phenolic extract represses hepatic inflammation in mice following alcohol-induced liver injury via inactivation of the hepatic endotoxin-TLR-4-NF-κB pathway (Xiao et al. 2020).

There is growing evidence that Biobran/MGN-3 is an effective therapeutic to complement conventional cancer treatment (Ooi et al. 2018). Moreover, dietary consumption of rice bran-derived AXs, including Biobran, has shown promising therapeutic effects in cancer patients including ameliorating cancer-associated inflammation. Kim et al. (2020) showed that patients undergoing cancer therapy alongside consumption of AX-rich fermented rice bran over an 8-week intervention had significantly ($P < 0.05$; $n = 10$) reduced levels of IL-1β and IL-6 secretion by LPS-stimulated peripheral blood mononuclear cells. In a rat model of liver carcinogenesis, treatment with Biobran inhibited inflammation and associated fibrosis by blocking liver cell expression of NF-κB (Badr El-Din et al. 2020). In unstimulated cells, NF-κB binds to its inhibitor IκB-α in the cytoplasm. When IκB-α becomes phosphorylated, NF-κB is released and becomes activated. The activated NF-κB then translocates to the nucleus where it acts as a transcription factor, stimulating the transcription of numerous pro-inflammatory genes. The hepatoprotective activity of Biobran in hepatocarcinogenic rats was correlated with both a reduction in inflammatory infiltrates and reversal of the carcinogen-induced degradation of IκB-α (Badr El-Din et al. 2020). Dokkaew et al. (2019) showed rice bran extract blocks iNOS, TNF-α, and NF-κB expression in rats with early hepatocarcinogenesis. The ferulic acid component of rice AX has been shown to suppress COX-2 activity, phosphorylation of IκB-α, nuclear translocation of NF-κB, NOS-2 (iNOS) gene expression, and production of TNF-α and IL-6 in cancers (Desai et al. 2018).

Chronic neuroinflammation has been observed in a number of brain diseases, including Parkinson's disease, Alzheimer's disease, schizophrenia, and depression (Kurtys et al. 2018). Biobran/MGN-3 has been shown by Ghoneum and El Sayed (2021) to be protective against sporadic Alzheimer's disease in mice, with Biobran treatment showing decreased levels of IL-6 and ICAM-1. Peripheral inflammatory conditions, such as colitis or LPS–induced sepsis, have been shown to activate microglia and initiate neuroinflammation (Chen et al. 2012; Riazi et al. 2008). The anti-inflammatory effects of rice bran fibres on neuroinflammation have been widely described (Kurtys et al. 2018). Abd El Fattah et al. (2021) showed rice bran can protect against LPS-induced neuroinflammation in a murine model by activating peroxisome proliferator-activated receptor-gamma (PPAR-γ) nuclear receptor. Bhatia et al. (2016) showed rice bran blocked prostaglandin release in LPS-activated primary microglia via reduced COX-2 and microsomal prostaglandin E synthase-1 (mPGES-1). Rice bran inhibited microglial activation by interfering with MAPK signalling and blocking the IkB-α degradation observed in LPS-activated microglia, leading to enhanced microglial production of the anti-inflammatory cytokine IL-10, and reduced the expression of pro-inflammatory markers TNF-α and IL-1β (Bhatia et al. 2016). Ferulic acid isolated from ferulated rice bran arabinoxylans through hydrolysis by bacterial enzymes provides neuroprotective and anti-neuroinflammatory effects in a murine model partly by reducing the levels of pro-inflammatory mediators, including TNF-α, IL-6, NF-κB, COX-2, and iNOS (Das et al. 2014).

Obesity and the development of type 2 diabetes due to insulin resistance is characterised by chronic, systemic low-grade inflammation in adipose tissue. Stabilised rice bran has been proposed as a potential treatment for diabetes due to its anti-inflammatory activities which include inhibition of COX-1, COX-2, and

5-lipooxygenase pro-inflammatory enzymes (Roschek et al. 2009). A rice bran-supplemented diet reverses the elevation of IL-1 β, TNF-α, IL-6, and iNOS observed in the adipose tissue of obese Zucker rats (Candiracci et al. 2014). Rice bran extract also reduced vascular inflammation in obese Zucker rats by reducing aortic superoxide levels, iNOS expression, and TNF-α production (Justo et al. 2013). Male Wistar rats fed a high-sugar and high-fat diet supplemented with rice bran, as shown by Siqueira et al. (2021), have reduced levels of renal inflammatory markers, including IL-6 and TNF-α. In obese mice on a high-fat diet, rice bran supplementation significantly ($P < 0.05$; $n = 6$) reduced myocardial COX-2 and matrix metalloproteinase-9 (MMP-9) activity, hepatic and serum TNF-α levels, and hepatic and heart NF-κB expression (Duansak et al. 2020). Moreover, the mRNA expression of IL-1β and IL-6 in white adipose tissue was significantly reduced in obese mice on high-fat diets supplemented with rice bran (Justo et al. 2016). In a human randomised controlled trial involving overweight and obese subjects placed on an energy-restricted diet, consumption of rice bran significantly reduced the pro-inflammatory markers CRP and IL-6 compared to the control group lacking rice bran treatment (Edrisi et al. 2018).

In a randomised controlled trial involving 40 patients, Biobran/MGN-3 treatment for 4 weeks reduced the low-grade inflammation associated with irritable bowel syndrome (IBS), and this anti-inflammatory effect was mirrored by a reduction in the inflammatory marker CRP (Kamiya et al. 2014). In a murine model of colitis, the anti-inflammatory activity of ferulic acid from rice bran was mediated through inhibition of NF-κB activity (Islam et al. 2008). Fermented rice bran has also been shown to reduce myeloperoxidase, IL-1β, IL-6, IL-17, and TNF-α in a murine model of colitis (Islam et al. 2017). MGN-3 arabinoxylan has been shown by Zhao et al. (2020) to reduce IL-1β, TNF-α, IL-6, and IL-8 levels in the serum and jejunal/colonic mucosa of male mice following radiation-induced intestinal injury.

The chronic inflammation associated with atherosclerosis has been shown to be reversed by dietary supplementation of rice bran extract, leading to reduced gene expression of aortic (TNF-α, IL-1β, iNOS) and hepatic (TNF-α, IL-1α, IL-1β) inflammatory markers (Tan et al. 2020). Furthermore, Tan et al. (2020) revealed that LPS-stimulated gene expression of iNOS, TNF-α, IL-1α, IL-1β, and IL-6 in J774A.1 macrophage-like cells was ameliorated following treatment with the rice bran extract. The anti-inflammatory effect of rice bran extract on atherosclerotic plaque development in obese mice on a high-fat diet may in part be due to reduced inflammatory cell infiltration (Perez-Ternero et al. 2017). In a rabbit model of atherosclerosis, treatment of hypercholesterolemic rabbits with rice bran from Njavara rice switched Janus kinase 2/signal transducer and activator of transcription 3 (JAK2-STAT3) activation in macrophages, leading to an anti-inflammatory environment with increased IL-10 expression and reduced levels of IL-1β and CRP (Chithra et al. 2017).

In summary, there is accumulating evidence that rice bran extracts have profound effects on mediating inflammation (Fig. 4.1a). However, many of these rice bran extracts are poorly characterised, and it is often difficult to ascertain which constituent(s) of the extract are contributing to the observed anti-inflammatory effects in previously published works. Despite this drawback, research specifically investigating rice bran AXs or AX-derived constituents is gradually developing in the literature, highlighting some common patterns (mediators) of anti-inflammatory activity mediated by rice bran AXs (Fig. 4.1b) or AX-derived compounds such as ferulic acid and feruloylated oligosaccharides (Fig. 4.1c). The body of published anti-inflammatory research on rice bran AX mostly focuses on utilising Biobran/ MGN-3, which highlights the potential scope to investigate a wider range of non-modified rice bran AXs in the future to complement the extensive work conducted on MGN-3. Application of the emerging anti-inflammatory properties of rice bran AXs as a potential treatment or prophylactic therapy for a wide range of inflammatory diseases is an exciting prospect that warrants further investigation.

References

Abd El Fattah MA, Abdelhamid YA, Elyamany MF, Badary OA, Heikal OA (2021) Rice bran extract protected against LPS-induced neuroinflammation in mice through targeting PPAR-γ nuclear receptor. Mol Neurobiol 58:1504–1516

Akihisa T, Yasukawa K, Yamaura M, Ukiya M, Kimura Y, Shimizu N et al (2000) Triterpene alcohol and sterol ferulates from rice bran and their anti-inflammatory effects. J Agric Food Chem 48:2313–2319

Badr El-Din NK, Ali DA, Othman R, French SW, Ghoneum M (2020) Chemopreventive role of arabinoxylan rice bran, MGN-3/Biobran, on liver carcinogenesis in rats. Biomed Pharmacother 126:110064

Bhatia HS, Baron J, Hagl S, Eckert GP, Fiebich BL (2016) Rice bran derivatives alleviate microglia activation: possible involvement of MAPK pathway. J Neuroinflammation 13:148

BioBran Research Foundation (2013) BioBran/MGN-3 (Rice bran arabinoxylan compound): basic and clinical application to integrative medicine, 2nd edn. BioBran Research Foundation, Tokyo

Broekaert WF, Courtin CM, Verbeke K, Van de Wiele T, Verstraete W, Delcour JA (2011) Prebiotic and other health-related effects of cereal-derived arabinoxylans, arabinoxylan-oligosaccharides, and xylooligosaccharides. Crit Rev Food Sci Nutr 51:178–194

Candiracci M, Justo ML, Castaño A, Rodriguez-Rodriguez R, Herrera MD (2014) Rice bran enzymatic extract-supplemented diets modulate adipose tissue inflammation markers in Zucker rats. Nutrition 30:466–472

Chen Z, Jalabi W, Shpargel KB, Farabaugh KT, Dutta R, Yin X et al (2012) Lipopolysaccharide-induced microglial activation and neuroprotection against experimental brain injury is independent of hematogenous TLR4. J Neurosci 32:11706–11715

Chithra PK, Jayalekshmy A, Helen A (2017) Petroleum ether extract of Njavara rice (Oryza sativa) bran upregulates the JAK2-STAT3-mediated anti-inflammatory profile in macrophages and aortic endothelial cells promoting regression of atherosclerosis. Biochem Cell Biol 95:652–662

Choi SP, Kim SP, Kang MY, Nam SH, Friedman M (2010) Protective effects of black rice bran against chemically-induced inflammation of mouse skin. J Agric Food Chem 58:10007–10015

Cholujova D, Jakubikova J, Sedlak J (2009) BioBran-augmented maturation of human monocyte-derived dendritic cells. Neoplasma 56:89–95

Cholujova D, Jakubikova J, Czako B, Martisova M, Hunakova L, Duraj J et al (2013) MGN-3 arabinoxylan rice bran modulates innate immunity in multiple myeloma patients. Cancer Immunol Immunother 62:437–445

Das U, Manna K, Sinha M, Datta S, Das DK, Chakraborty A et al (2014) Role of ferulic acid in the amelioration of ionizing radiation induced inflammation: a murine model. PLoS One 9:e97599

Desai SJ, Prickril B, Rasooly A (2018) Mechanisms of phytonutrient modulation of cyclooxygenase-2 (cox-2) and inflammation related to cancer. Nutr Cancer 70:350–375

Dokkaew A, Punvittayagul C, Insuan O, Limtrakul Dejkriengkraikul P, Wongpoomchai R (2019) Protective effects of defatted sticky rice bran extracts on the early stages of hepatocarcinogenesis in rats. Molecules 24:2142

Duansak N, Piyabhan P, Srisawat U, Naowaboot J, Lerdvuthisopon N, Schmid-Schönbein G (2020) The effect of rice bran extract on arterial blood pressure, hepatic steatosis, and inflammation in mice fed with a high-fat diet. J Nutr Metab 2020:8374287

Edrisi F, Salehi M, Ahmadi A, Fararoei M, Rusta F, Mahmoodianfard S (2018) Effects of supplementation with rice husk powder and rice bran on inflammatory factors in overweight and obese adults following an energy-restricted diet: a randomized controlled trial. Eur J Nutr 57:833–843

Elsaid AF, Shaheen M, Ghoneum M (2018) Biobran/MGN-3, an arabinoxylan rice bran, enhances NK cell activity in geriatric subjects: a randomized, double-blind, placebo-controlled clinical trial. Exp Ther Med 15:2313–2320

Fadel A, Mahmoud AM, Ashworth JJ, Li W, Ng YL, Plunkett A (2018a) Health-related effects and improving extractability of cereal arabinoxylans. Int J Biol Macromol 109:819–831

Fadel A, Plunkett A, Li W, Tessu Gyamfi VE, Nyaranga RR, Fadel F et al (2018b) Modulation of innate and adaptive immune responses by arabinoxylans. J Food Biochem 42:e12473

Fan JP, Choi KM, Han GD (2010) Inhibitory effects of water extracts of fermented rice bran on allergic response. Food Sci Biotechnol 19:1573–1578

Fang H-Y, Chen Y-K, Chen H-H, Lin S-Y, Fang Y-T (2012) Immunomodulatory effects of feruloylated oligosaccharides from rice bran. Food Chem 134:836–840

Friedman M (2013) Rice brans, rice bran oils, and rice hulls: composition, food and industrial uses, and bioactivities in humans, animals, and cells. J Agric Food Chem 61:10626–10641

Ghoneum M (1998) Anti-HIV activity in vitro of MGN-3, an activated arabinoxylane from rice bran. Biochem Biophys Res Commun 243:25–29

Ghoneum M, Abedi S (2004) Enhancement of natural killer cell activity of aged mice by modified arabinoxylan rice bran (MGN-3/Biobran). J Pharm Pharmacol 56:1581–1588

Ghoneum M, Agrawal S (2011) Activation of human monocyte-derived dendritic cells in vitro by the biological response modifier arabinoxylan rice bran (MGN-3/Biobran). Int J Immunopathol Pharmacol 24:941–948

Ghoneum MH, El Sayed NS (2021) Protective effect of Biobran/MGN-3 against sporadic Alzheimer's disease mouse model: possible role of oxidative stress and apoptotic pathways. Oxidative Med Cell Longev 2021:8845064

Ghoneum M, Gollapudi S (2003) Modified arabinoxylan rice bran (MGN-3/Biobran) sensitizes human T cell leukemia cells to death receptor (CD95)-induced apoptosis. Cancer Lett 201:41–49

Ghoneum M, Matsuura M (2004) Augmentation of macrophage phagocytosis by modified arabinoxylan rice bran (MGN-3/Biobran). Int J Immunopathol Pharmacol 17:283–292

Ghoneum M, Matsuura M, Gollapudi S (2008) Modified arabinoxylan rice bran (Mgn-3/Biobran) enhances intracellular killing of microbes by human phagocytic cells in vitro. Int J Immunopathol Pharmacol 21:87–95

Hoshino Y, Hirashima N, Nakanishi M, Furuno T (2010) Inhibition of degranulation and cytokine production in bone marrow-derived mast cells by hydrolyzed rice bran. Inflamm Res 59:615–625

Ichihashi K (2004) Experience with administration of BioBran in patients with chronic rheumatism. Clin Pharmacol Ther 14:459–463

Islam MS, Murata T, Fujisawa M, Nagasaka R, Ushio H, Bari AM et al (2008) Anti-inflammatory effects of phytosteryl ferulates in colitis induced by dextran sulphate sodium in mice. Br J Pharmacol 154:812–824

Islam MS, Nagasaka R, Ohara K, Hosoya T, Ozaki H, Ushio H et al (2011) Biological abilities of rice bran-derived antioxidant phytochemicals for medical therapy. Curr Top Med Chem 11: 1847–1853

Islam J, Koseki T, Watanabe K, Budijanto S, Oikawa A, Alauddin M et al (2017) Dietary supplementation of fermented rice bran effectively alleviates dextran sodium sulfate-induced colitis in mice. Nutrients 9:747

Ji MG, Lee YR, Nam YH, Castañeda R, Hong BN, Kang TH (2020) Immunostimulatory action of high-content active arabinoxylan in rice bran. ACS Omega 5:26374–26381

Jun H-I, Shin J-W, Song G-S, Kim Y-S (2015) Isolation and identification of phenolic antioxidants in black rice bran. J Food Sci 80:C262–C268

Justo ML, Candiracci M, Dantas AP, de Sotomayor MA, Parrado J, Vila E et al (2013) Rice bran enzymatic extract restores endothelial function and vascular contractility in obese rats by reducing vascular inflammation and oxidative stress. J Nutr Biochem 24:1453–1461

Justo ML, Claro C, Zeyda M, Stulnig TM, Herrera MD, Rodríguez-Rodríguez R (2016) Rice bran prevents high-fat diet-induced inflammation and macrophage content in adipose tissue. Eur J Nutr 55:2011–2019

Kamiya T, Shikano M, Tanaka M, Ozeki K, Ebi M, Katano T et al (2014) Therapeutic effects of biobran, modified arabinoxylan rice bran, in improving symptoms of diarrhea predominant or mixed type irritable bowel syndrome: a pilot, randomized controlled study. Evid Based Complement Alternat Med 2014:828137

Kang H, Lee M-G, Lee J-K, Choi Y-H, Choi Y-S (2016) Enzymatically-processed wheat bran enhances macrophage activity and has in vivo anti-inflammatory effects in mice. Nutrients 8: 188

Kim H-Y, Park J, Lee K-H, Lee D-U, Kwak J-H, Kim YS et al (2011) Ferulic acid protects against carbon tetrachloride-induced liver injury in mice. Toxicology 282:104–111

Kim J-M, Hong S-G, Song B-S, Sohn H-J, Baik H, Sung M-K (2020) Efficacy of cereal-based oral nutrition supplement on nutritional status, inflammatory cytokine secretion and quality of life in cancer patients under cancer therapy. J Cancer Prev 25:55–63

Kurtys E, Eisel ULM, Hageman RJJ, Verkuyl JM, Broersen LM, Dierckx RAJO et al (2018) Anti-inflammatory effects of rice bran components. Nutr Rev 76:372–379

Lee S-H, Seo MJ, Choi SM, Sohn YS, Kang KK, Ahn BO et al (2005) DA-9201 shows anti-asthmatic effects by suppressing NF-kappaB expression in an ovalbumin-induced mouse model of asthma. Arch Pharm Res 28:1350–1357

Lee CY, Lee MJ, Kim JM, Choi SM, Kang KK, Kim OJ et al (2015) Oryza sativa L. extracts inhibit nitric oxide production and inducible nitric oxide synthase expression in murine macrophage cells and lungs of antigen-challenged allergic mice. Int J Phytomed 7:1–7

Lee A, Ko J, Ahn S-J, Joo Kim H, Min S-S, Kim E (2021) Potential effects of pigmented rice on immunity: a review focusing on anthocyanins, gamma-oryzanol, and arabinoxylan. J Food Nutr Res 9:26–31

Mendis M, Leclerc E, Simsek S (2016) Arabinoxylan hydrolyzates as immunomodulators in lipopolysaccharide-induced RAW264.7 macrophages. Food Funct 7:3039–3045

North CJ, Venter CS, Jerling JC (2009) The effects of dietary fibre on C-reactive protein, an inflammation marker predicting cardiovascular disease. Eur J Clin Nutr 63:921–933

Ogawa K, Takeuchi M, Nakamura N (2005) Immunological effects of partially hydrolyzed arabinoxylan from corn husk in mice. Biosci Biotechnol Biochem 69:19–25

Ooi SL, McMullen D, Golombick T, Pak SC (2018) Evidence-based review of BioBran/MGN-3 arabinoxylan compound as a complementary therapy for conventional cancer treatment. Integr Cancer Ther 17:165–178

Perez-Ternero C, Claro C, Parrado J, Herrera MD, Alvarez de Sotomayor M (2017) Rice bran enzymatic extract reduces atherosclerotic plaque development and steatosis in high-fat fed ApoE-/- mice. Nutrition 37:22–29

Riazi K, Galic MA, Kuzmiski JB, Ho W, Sharkey KA, Pittman QJ (2008) Microglial activation and TNFalpha production mediate altered CNS excitability following peripheral inflammation. Proc Natl Acad Sci U S A 105:17151–17156

Roschek BJ, Fink RC, Li D, McMichael M, Tower CM, Smith RD et al (2009) Pro-inflammatory enzymes, cyclooxygenase 1, cyclooxygenase 2, and 5-lipooxygenase, inhibited by stabilized rice bran extracts. J Med Food 12:615–623

Saji N, Francis N, Blanchard CL, Schwarz LJ, Santhakumar AB (2019) Rice bran phenolic compounds regulate genes associated with antioxidant and anti-inflammatory activity in human umbilical vein endothelial cells with induced oxidative stress. Int J Mol Sci 20:4715

Saji N, Francis N, Schwarz LJ, Blanchard CL, Santhakumar AB (2020) The antioxidant and anti-inflammatory properties of rice bran phenolic extracts. Foods 9:829

Sakai S, Ochiai H, Nakajima K, Terasawa K (1997) Inhibitory effect of ferulic acid on macrophage inflammatory protein-2 production in a murine macrophage cell line, RAW264.7. Cytokine 9: 242–248

Sharif MK, Butt MS, Anjum FM, Khan SH (2014) Rice bran: a novel functional ingredient. Crit Rev Food Sci Nutr 54:807–816

Siqueira JS, Francisqueti-Ferron FV, Garcia JL, de Almeida Silva CCV, Costa MR, Nakandakare-Maia ET et al (2021) Rice bran modulates renal disease risk factors in animals submitted to high sugar-fat diet. Brazilian. J Nephrol 43:156–164

Tan XW, Kobayashi K, Shen L, Inagaki J, Ide M, Hwang SS et al (2020) Antioxidative attributes of rice bran extracts in ameliorative effects of atherosclerosis-associated risk factors. Heliyon 6: e05743

Udani J, Hardy ML (2006) Rice bran arabinoxylan for regulation of the immune system. Integr Med Alert 9:125–128

Webber DM, Hettiarachchy NS, Li R, Horax R, Theivendran S (2014) Phenolic profile and antioxidant activity of extracts prepared from fermented heat-stabilized defatted rice bran. J Food Sci 79:H2383–H2391

Xiao J, Zhang R, Wu Y, Wu C, Jia X, Dong L et al (2020) Rice bran phenolic extract protects against alcoholic liver injury in mice by alleviating intestinal microbiota dysbiosis, barrier dysfunction, and liver inflammation mediated by the endotoxin-tlr4-nf-κb pathway. J Agric Food Chem 68:1237–1247

Zhang S, Li W, Smith CJ, Musa H (2015) Cereal-derived arabinoxylans as biological response modifiers: extraction, molecular features, and immune-stimulating properties. Crit Rev Food Sci Nutr 55:1035–1052

Zhao Z, Cheng W, Qu W, Wang K (2020) Arabinoxylan rice bran (MGN-3/Biobran) alleviates radiation-induced intestinal barrier dysfunction of mice in a mitochondrion-dependent manner. Biomed Pharmacother 124:109855

Zheng S, Sugita S, Hirai S, Egashira Y (2012a) Protective effect of low molecular fraction of MGN-3, a modified arabinoxylan from rice bran, on acute liver injury by inhibition of NF-κB and JNK/MAPK expression. Int Immunopharmacol 14:764–769

Zheng S, Sanada H, Dohi H, Hirai S, Egashira Y (2012b) Suppressive effect of modified arabinoxylan from rice bran (MGN-3) on D-galactosamine-induced IL-18 expression and hepatitis in rats. Biosci Biotechnol Biochem 76:942–946

Part III

Applications in Cancer

Part III aims at detailing the therapeutic applications of RBAC in cancer. Scientific evidence for the use of RBAC as a supporting treatment for cancer will be explored.

Integrative Oncology 5

Romulo Jacinto S. de Villa

Abstract

Integrative oncology is a branch of integrative medicine that combines the treatment of cancer patients with complementary and conventional modalities. It aims to enhance the effect of conventional treatments and optimize the quality of life and emotional health of cancer patients. Carcinogenesis involves the transformation of normal cells into cancer cells through random damage to control genes, leading to uncontrolled growth, proliferation, and invasion of cancer cells into normal tissues. While chemotherapy and bio-targeted therapy address cancer spread from the initial tumor, surgery and radiotherapy deal with the growing mass, and immunotherapy addresses those cancer cells that knock out the immune system's ability to recognize them. Conventional cancer management targets early-stage cancer with curative intent and late-stage cancer with palliative intent. Complementary modalities in cancer management encompass mind/body practices, natural products, and lifestyle modification. When diet therapy and nutraceutical medicine are used in cancer management, it is referred to as nutritional oncology. Modified rice bran arabinoxylan is a nutraceutical that has been shown to improve the quality of life in breast cancer patients, reduce the chemotherapy side effects, enhance the response rate to chemotherapy in liver cancer, provide radioprotective effects in cervical cancer, augment immunity in multiple myeloma, and prolong survival of patients in many case studies. Integrative oncology has emerged as a new field of medical practice to improve cancer patients' survival and quality of life.

R. J. S. de Villa (✉)
National Kidney and Transplant Institute, Quezon City, Metro Manila, Philippines

S. C. Pak et al. (eds.), *Modified Rice Bran Arabinoxylan*,
https://doi.org/10.1007/978-981-19-5735-2_5

Keywords

Integrative medicine · Complementary therapy · Natural products · Lifestyle modification · Nutritional oncology · Evidence-based integration

5.1 Definition of Integrative Oncology

Integrative oncology is a branch of integrative medicine, which combines complementary medicine modalities with conventional medicine. Integrative oncology focuses on the treatment of cancer patients with complementary and conventional modalities. Conventional modalities for cancer treatment include surgery, radiotherapy, chemotherapy, targeted biotherapies, and immunotherapy. The complementary modalities include mind and body practices, natural products, and lifestyle modifications.

Integrative oncology emerged as a response to cancer patients' desire for holistic care (Leis et al. 2008). Cancer patients often request care that not only focuses on treating their disease but also takes into consideration the source of their illness, optimizes their health, and enhances their well-being. Based on the increasing evidence for the safety and effectiveness of many complementary modalities in cancer care, several hospitals and medical centers apply these complementary modalities to meet cancer patients' needs (Cramer et al. 2013; Grant et al. 2019).

Integrative oncology is a relatively new field. A comprehensive consensus definition has been developed, which states, "Integrative Oncology is a patient-centered, evidence-informed field of cancer care that utilizes mind and body practices, natural products, and/or lifestyle modifications from different traditions alongside conventional cancer treatments. Integrative Oncology aims to optimize health, quality of life, and clinical outcomes across the cancer care continuum and to empower people to prevent cancer and become active participants before, during, and beyond cancer treatment" (Witt et al. 2017).

5.2 The Principle of Integration in Cancer Patient Management

To understand the principle of integration, we must understand carcinogenesis in the patient's body. Carcinogenesis involves the process of initiation, promotion, and progression (Yamagiwa and Ichikawa 1918). Initiation involves random damage to genes. Promotion involves stimulation of uncontrolled growth and proliferation of cells either directly or indirectly by causing inflammation. During inflammation, several growth factors are released. Hence, chronic inflammation is a factor in developing and progressing or worsening cancers (Coussens and Werb 2002). Progression involves the development of more aggressive, destructive, and more invasive behavior of cancer cells.

Initiators damage genes that control the behavior of a cell. When multiple control points within a cell have been damaged, the cell will lose control and continually perform that behavior. When a cell loses control of growth and proliferation, the cell becomes a tumor or a growing mass of cells. Surgery and radiotherapy are treatments that address this growing mass of cells.

This uncontrolled cell behavior is passed on to the succeeding generation of cells because damaged genes are copied or duplicated during cell growth prior to proliferation. Thus, when an initiator damaged the genes, a normal cell is transformed into a tumor cell. When genes controlling the behavior of mobility and invasiveness are damaged, then the tumor cell transforms into a cancer cell (Cooper and Hausman 2013). Chemotherapy and bio-targeted therapy address cancer that has spread out from the initial tumor mass.

Continuous exposure to initiators will lead to further disease progression because additional behavior controlling genes may be damaged. A variety of behaviors emerge in the different cancer cells enabling them to become intelligent for survival. Diet and lifestyle modification can reduce the load of initiators entering the body and moderate their survival intelligence.

Cancer cells induce branching of blood vessels that extend to the tumor mass, providing nutrition even to the cancer cells in the inner regions of the mass. This ability enables cancer to grow into a larger mass. Surgery and radiotherapy can address this growing mass. There are targeted therapies and natural products that can block cancer cells' ability to make blood vessels grow.

There are cancer cells that knock out the immune system's ability to recognize them (Cornel et al. 2020). Immunotherapy will address these kinds of cancer cells. Physical activity lifestyle modification helps improve immunity. Some cancer cells make the immune surveillance blind. There are natural products that can bring back immune recognition of cancer cells. Certain cancer cells camouflage themselves from the immune system while traveling in the blood, going to distant areas of the body. There are natural products that can dissolve the camouflage.

There are cancer cells that induce muscle protein breakdown into amino acids. There are cancer cells that make the liver produce glucose from amino acids. There are oral nutritional supplements that can block these abilities of cancer cells.

Initiators include ionizing radiation that damages genes, infectious agents that disrupt control genes, and mostly human-made pollutant chemicals that damage and kill cells. Pollution is a major factor that has influenced the development of cancer. These initiator pollutants accumulate in some geographical regions where polluted waters gather, such as rivers, river mouths, shallow waters of the sea, and animals higher up in the food chain. Processing of foods adds more initiator chemicals into the food supply, such as in processed red meats (Santarelli et al. 2008). Thus, it is advisable to avoid processed red meats and reduce red meat consumption to reduce cancer risk.

Promoters allow the accumulation of multiple genes to be damaged, which shortens the time it takes for the cell to lose control of its behavior. That is why targeting a single gene defect in the behavior control pathways is usually not sufficient. Multiple control points must be targeted to stop uncontrolled behavior.

Chemotherapy is usually more effective in combination with other chemotherapy drugs and bio-targeted therapies (Bayat Mokhtari et al. 2017).

Another factor that comes into play in a patient with cancer is stress. Stress increases cortisol levels, which increases the liver production of glucose and lowers immunity. Glucose feeds cancer with energy and materials for its growth. Weakened immunity allows cancer to escape. The complementary modality of mind and body practices has been shown to reduce the stress level (Kim et al. 2013).

5.3 Role of Conventional Modalities in Cancer Management

Cancer cells continuously and uncontrollably grow and proliferate or multiply in numbers. They increase in numbers exponentially. By the time cancer is symptomatic, detected, and diagnosed, their number is already in the billions. Thus, the fight against cancer is a numbers game. To treat cancer, it may be required to drastically reduce cancer cell numbers, which is the role of conventional therapies such as surgery, radiotherapy, chemotherapy, bio-targeted therapy, and immunotherapy.

The conventional management of cancer utilizes treatment modalities wherein their effectiveness is supported with clinical studies reaching the level of a double-blind, randomized controlled clinical trial (RCT) on hundreds of subjects, even thousands. Conventional medicine modalities have well-described adverse reactions or side effects, which are often managed.

The conventional treatment modalities are designed to treat early-stage (stages 0, I, and II) cancer with curative intent and late-stage (stages III and IV) and terminal diseases with palliative intent slowing down cancer growth. In the past, cancer was grouped into the early and late stages. Cancer is currently grouped into metastatic and nonmetastatic disease wherein stage IV is metastatic disease and stages I, II, and III are nonmetastatic disease (American Cancer Society 2020).

The roles of surgery in cancer patient management include (Canadian Cancer Society 2020):

1. Obtain tissue for diagnosis and staging.
2. Remove very early stage of cancer to achieve a possible cure.
3. Relieve the symptoms of a large cancer tumor.
4. Remove sites of recurrence.
5. Reconstruct tissue damaged by cancer.
6. Prevent cancer in high-risk individuals.

The role of chemotherapy is to reduce the number of cancer cells that have spread throughout the body and prolong cancer patient survival (Lee et al. 2018). The role of bio-targeted therapy is to target specific genes and proteins involved in cancer cells' growth and survival, affecting the tissue environment of cancer cells or target cells related to cancer growth like blood vessel cells (Cancer.Net Editorial Board 2020a). The role of immunotherapy is for cancer cells to be recognized and targeted by the body's immune system and prolong survival (Cancer Research Institute 2020).

5.4 Role of Complementary Modalities in Cancer Management

5.4.1 Mind and Body Practices

Mind and body practices are not therapeutic, but they address a person's well-being, quality of life, pain, and energy. The modality of mind and body practices include hypnosis (mind), relaxation techniques (mind), talk therapy, meditation, visualization, music therapy, art therapy, aromatherapy, qigong (body and mind), acupuncture (body), reflexology (body), and massage therapy (body).

Stress feeds cancer due to cortisol, the stress hormone, causing the liver to produce glucose (Lecavalier et al. 1990), and lower immunity (Brzozowski et al. 2016). Thus, mind and body practices such as relaxation techniques, meditation, and yoga help reduce stress hormone levels and improve immunity (Smith 2013).

The states of mind and body influence the immune system, which defends the body from cancer. Regular moderate exercise enhances immunosurveillance and may help reduce the risk of cancer (Nieman and Pence 2020). Mind and body practices also improve salivary immunoglobulin A levels and positively affect immune outcomes (Wahbeh et al. 2009).

5.4.2 Natural Products

Natural products include dietary supplements, herbal medicine, and nutraceuticals. Natural products:

1. Assist conventional treatment modalities in killing cancer cells by apoptosis, starving cancer from growing its blood supply, and supporting the functionality of the immune system.
2. Help protect healthy normal cells from collateral damage from conventional treatments.
3. Block the ability of cancer cells to feed on the body.

5.4.2.1 Dietary Supplements

People with cancer take dietary supplements in an attempt to be cured of cancer. A dietary supplement is any vitamin, mineral, botanical/plant-derived material, enzymes, amino acids, or other dietary ingredients taken by mouth and added to a diet. In the United States, it is not required to prove safety or efficacy when a dietary supplement is registered with the Food and Drug Administration. The only requirement is to place a label stating, "No Approved Therapeutic Claim" (Dwyer et al. 2018).

5.4.2.2 Herbal Medicine

Herbal medicine can be considered traditional or modern (Wikipedia 2020). Traditional herbal medicine is also called phytotherapy, which involves crude plant preparations, whereas modern herbal medicine is purified extracts with clinical trials on safety and efficacy. Modern herbal medicine is part of a class of natural products called nutraceutical medicine. Herbal medicine may have a role in the mitigation of reactive oxygen species and autophagy in cancer therapy (Marzvanyan et al. 2018).

5.4.2.3 Nutraceutical Medicine, Natural Product Drugs, and Botanical Drugs

The field of nutraceuticals is another emerging area with various definitions. Stephen de Felice initially coined the word nutraceuticals from "nutrition" and "pharmaceuticals." He defined it as food or parts of food that provide medical or health benefits, including preventing and treating disease (Kalra 2003). In the form of food, the nutraceutical is aptly called a functional food. Another term could be nutraceutical medicine, which would be defined as a natural product

1. Obtained from mostly plants and herbs.
2. Formulated into powder or liquid placed in capsule, sachet, or tablet form.
3. Evaluated for safety and efficacy in human clinical trials.

Other terms used that fall within this definition of nutraceutical medicine are natural product drugs or botanical drugs. Nutraceuticals are a marketing term, while botanical drugs and natural product drugs are terms used by regulatory authorities. Nutraceuticals are registered as dietary supplements, while natural product drugs and botanical drugs are registered as drugs.

One of the major sources of drug discovery is from plants (Katiyar et al. 2012). Plant herbs have been the source of compounds converted into evidence-based pharmaceutical drugs called botanical drugs. There is increasing use of botanical drugs globally, growing annually by 8–10% (Ahn 2017). Proper double-blind controlled clinical trials are needed to determine plants' safety and efficacy before they can be recommended for medical use (Vickers 2007).

These nutraceutical medicines, natural product drugs, or botanical drugs are:

1. Extracted from nature (although the purity may be low, moderate, or high. Some products reach as high as 97% purity (Grkovic et al. 2020). However, there will be no nature-derived compound that will reach 100% equivalence to a synthetic drug).
2. Purified to obtain the active compound (although there are extracts where the active compound has not been identified).
3. Standardized to contain a consistent amount of active compound (amount of active compounds found in plants varies based on the climate conditions, available nutrients in the soil, and plant variety).
4. Studied for safety to the human body.

5. Studied for efficacy in the therapy of diseases and healthy structure and function of the human body.

5.5 Lifestyle Modification as a Complementary Modality

The role of lifestyle modifications is to:

1. Reduce the risk of cancer, which is increased by an unhealthy diet and lack of physical activity.
2. Support the nutritional needs of the patient without supporting the nutrition of cancer cells.
3. Enhance muscle strength and body fitness, which cancer weakens.

Malnutrition is a hallmark of cancer. Patients must recover from their poor nutritional status, which comes from cancer grabbing nutrients from the body. For example, cancer can utilize glucose more than normal cells because it makes the body relatively resistant to insulin (Dev et al. 2018). When a patient is told to eat and eat more of anything, glucose from the food feeds cancer more than the normal cells. Between the three sources of energy, carbohydrates, fats, and proteins, cancer prefers glucose, as evidenced by the use of labeled glucose to detect cancer in positron emission tomography and computerized tomography scans (Croteau et al. 2016). We must find a way to starve cancer from its energy source without starving the body.

5.5.1 Nutritional Oncology

Nutritional oncology is the use of diet therapy and nutraceutical medicine/botanical drugs in cancer management. In nutritional oncology, there is a way to feed the patient without feeding cancer and starve cancer without starving the patient. Cancer cells exclusively derive energy from glucose and not from fats and proteins, while normal cells of the body can derive energy from carbohydrates, fats, and even proteins. If the patient reduces or stops eating carbohydrates and eats mostly fats and proteins, cancer will be starved of energy, but not the patient's body. Currently, there are numerous clinical trials on dietary interventions for cancer therapy (Lévesque et al. 2019).

5.5.2 Physical Activity

Studies suggest that doing any kind of physical activity that reduces sitting can help lower cancer risk (Cancer.Net Editorial Board 2020b). Regular exercise within one's limit improves physical and mental health during conventional cancer treatment (Cancer.Net Editorial Board 2020c).

5.6 Evidence-Based Integration

There is a need for studies to support integrating complementary modalities with conventional cancer patient management collaboratively and synergistically.

RCTs are the "gold standard" in clinical research because of the strong inherent validity emanating from the design's ability to control bias, confounding factors, and error. However, for studies of complementary therapies in integrative oncology, the validity of RCT may not be possible to achieve for many of the complementary modalities. For natural products, like nutraceuticals that can be standardized as to the amount of active component, RCTs can be performed. These studies' outcome measures may be objective such as survival data or response rates or subjective such as patient desires (e.g., pain control, improved capacity for daily living, quality of life). However, these studies usually have only small sample sizes because RCTs are costly, and natural products cannot be patented. Another company can simply use the results of the study to market the same natural product.

One of the nutraceuticals that advanced to RCT level is modified rice bran arabinoxylan (BioBran/MGN-3/Lentin plus). In a review paper (Ooi et al. 2018), rice bran arabinoxylan has been shown to:

1. Improve the quality of life in breast cancer patients (Masood et al. 2013).
2. Reduce the chemotherapy side effects in breast cancer (Masood et al. 2013) and a variety of cancers (Petrovics et al. 2016).
3. Improve the response rate to chemotherapy in hepatocellular carcinoma (Bang et al. 2010).
4. Provide radioprotective effects in cervical cancer (Itoh et al. 2015).
5. Improve immunity in multiple myeloma (Cholujova et al. 2013).
6. Prolong survival in hepatocellular carcinoma and various cancers (Takahara and Sano 2004).

There is an ongoing trial on rice bran arabinoxylan's effect on the quality of life of cancer patients (Ooi et al. 2020).

Below are a few of the integrative oncology clinical trials integrating diet, vitamins, and natural products with conventional therapies.

1. A phase III study of ascorbic acid infusions combined with FOLFOX ± bevacizumab versus treatment with FOLFOX ± alone as first-line therapy in patients with recurrent or advanced colorectal cancer (Xu 2019).
2. How well the combination of ketogenic diet and chemotherapy works together to influence the return of cancer in patients with stage IV breast cancer (Volek 2018).
3. Pilot study on ketogenic diet treatment adjunctive to radiation and chemotherapy for newly diagnosed glioblastoma (Mid-Atlantic Epilepsy and Sleep Center LLC 2014).

Integrative oncology has emerged as a new field of medical practice that addresses various patient concerns with both conventional and complementary modalities anchored in the principles of integration, each with its role to improve patient survival and quality of life.

References

Ahn K (2017) The worldwide trend of using botanical drugs and strategies for developing global drugs. BMB Rep 50:111–116

American Cancer Society (2020) Understanding advanced and metastatic cancer [Internet]. [cited 2020 Nov 30]. https://www.cancer.org/treatment/understanding-your-diagnosis/advanced-cancer/what-is.html

Bang MH, Van Riep T, Thinh NT, Song LH, Dung TT, Van Troung L et al (2010) Arabinoxylan rice bran (MGN-3) enhances the effects of interventional therapies for the treatment of hepatocellular carcinoma: a three-year randomized clinical trial. Anticancer Res 30:5145–5151

Bayat Mokhtari R, Homayouni TS, Baluch N, Morgatskaya E, Kumar S, Das B et al (2017) Combination therapy in combating cancer. Oncotarget 8:38022–38043

Brzozowski B, Mazur-Bialy A, Pajdo R, Kwiecien S, Bilski J, Zwolinska-Wcislo M et al (2016) Mechanisms by which stress affects the experimental and clinical inflammatory bowel disease (ibd): role of brain-gut axis. Curr Neuropharmacol 14:892–900

Canadian Cancer Society (2020) Surgery in cancer treatment [Internet]. [cited 2020 Nov 30]. https://www.cancer.ca/en/cancer-information/diagnosis-and-treatment/surgery

Cancer Research Institute (2020) Benefits of cancer immunotherapy [Internet]. [cited 2020 Nov 30]. https://www.cancerresearch.org/immunotherapy/why-immunotherapy

Cancer.Net Editorial Board (2020a) Understanding targeted therapy [Internet]. Cancer.net. [cited 2020 Nov 30]. https://www.cancer.net/navigating-cancer-care/how-cancer-treated/personalized-and-targeted-therapies/understanding-targeted-therapy

Cancer.Net Editorial Board (2020b) Physical activity and cancer risk [Internet]. Cancer.Net. [cited 2020 Nov 30]. https://www.cancer.net/navigating-cancer-care/prevention-and-healthy-living/physical-activity-and-cancer-risk

Cancer.Net Editorial Board (2020c) Exercise during cancer treatment [Internet]. Cancer.net. [cited 2020 Nov 30]. https://www.cancer.net/survivorship/healthy-living/exercise-during-cancer-treatment

Cholujova D, Jakubikova J, Czako B, Martisova M, Hunakova L, Duraj J et al (2013) MGN-3 arabinoxylan rice bran modulates innate immunity in multiple myeloma patients. Cancer Immunol Immunother 62:437–445

Cooper GM, Hausman RE (2013) The cell: a molecular approach, 6th edn. Sinauer Associates, Sunderland, MA

Cornel AM, Mimpen IL, Nierkens S (2020) MHC class I downregulation in cancer: underlying mechanisms and potential targets for cancer immunotherapy. Cancers (Basel) 12:1760

Coussens LM, Werb Z (2002) Inflammation and cancer. Nature 420:860–867

Cramer H, Cohen L, Dobos G, Witt CM (2013) Integrative oncology: best of both worlds-theoretical, practical, and research issues. Evid Based Complement Alternat Med 2013:383142

Croteau E, Renaud JM, Richard MA, Ruddy TD, Bénard F, DeKemp RA (2016) PET metabolic biomarkers for cancer. Biomark Cancer 8:61–69

Dev R, Bruera E, Dalal S (2018) Insulin resistance and body composition in cancer patients. Ann Oncol 29:ii18–ii26

Dwyer JT, Coates PM, Smith MJ (2018) Dietary supplements: regulatory challenges and research resources. Nutrients 10:41

Grant SJ, Marthick M, Lacey J (2019) Establishing an integrative oncology service in the Australian healthcare setting-the Chris O'Brien Lifehouse Hospital experience. Support Care Cancer 27: 2069–2076

Grkovic T, Akee RK, Thornburg CC, Trinh SK, Britt JR, Harris MJ et al (2020) National Cancer Institute (NCI) program for natural products discovery: rapid isolation and identification of biologically active natural products from the NCI prefractionated library. ACS Chem Biol 15: 1104–1114

Itoh Y, Mizuno M, Ikeda M, Nakahara R, Kubota S, Ito J et al (2015) A randomized, double-blind pilot trial of hydrolyzed rice bran versus placebo for radioprotective effect on acute gastroenteritis secondary to chemoradiotherapy in patients with cervical cancer. Evid Based Complement Alternat Med 2015:974390

Kalra EK (2003) Nutraceutical-definition and introduction. AAPS PharmSci 5:E25

Katiyar C, Gupta A, Kanjilal S, Katiyar S (2012) Drug discovery from plant sources: an integrated approach. Ayu 33:10–19

Kim SH, Schneider SM, Kravitz L, Mermier C, Burge MR (2013) Mind-body practices for posttraumatic stress disorder. J Investig Med 61:827–834

Lecavalier L, Bolli G, Gerich J (1990) Glucagon-cortisol interactions on glucose turnover and lactate gluconeogenesis in normal humans. Am J Physiol Metab 258:E569–E575

Lee SB, Sohn G, Kim J, Chung IY, Kim HJ, Ko BS et al (2018) Chronological improvement in survival of patients with breast cancer: a large-scale, single-center study. J Breast Cancer 21:70–79

Leis AM, Weeks LC, Verhoef MJ (2008) Principles to guide integrative oncology and the development of an evidence base. Curr Oncol 15(Suppl 2):s83–s87

Lévesque S, Pol JG, Ferrere G, Galluzzi L, Zitvogel L, Kroemer G (2019) Trial watch: dietary interventions for cancer therapy. Onco Targets Ther 8:1591878

Marzvanyan A, Chen V, Zhang B, Asatrian G (2018) Herbal medicine in the mitigation of reactive oxygen species, autophagy, and cancer: a review. Crit Rev Oncog 23:333–346

Masood AI, Sheikh R, Anwer RA (2013) "BIOBRAN MGN-3"; effect of reducing side effects of chemotherapy in breast cancer patients. Prof Med J 20:13–16

Mid-Atlantic Epilepsy and Sleep Center LLC (2014) Ketogenic diet treatment adjunctive to radiation and chemotherapy in glioblastoma multiforme: a pilot study (GBMXRT) [Internet]. ClinicalTrials.gov. [cited 2020 Nov 30]. https://clinicaltrials.gov/ct2/show/NCT02302235

Nieman DC, Pence BD (2020) Exercise immunology: future directions. J Sport Health Sci 9:432–445

Ooi SL, McMullen D, Golombick T, Pak SC (2018) Evidence-based review of BioBran/MGN-3 arabinoxylan compound as a complementary therapy for conventional cancer treatment. Integr Cancer Ther 17:165–178

Ooi SL, Pak SC, Micalos PS, Schupfer E, Zielinski R, Jeffries T et al (2020) Rice bran arabinoxylan compound and quality of life of cancer patients (RBAC-QoL): study protocol for a randomized pilot feasibility trial. Contemp Clin Trials Commun 19:100580

Petrovics G, Szigeti G, Hamvas S, Máté Á, Betlehem J, Hegyi G (2016) Controlled pilot study for cancer patients suffering from chronic fatigue syndrome due to chemotherapy treated with BioBran (MGN-3-Arabinoxylane) and targeted radiofrequency heat therapy. Eur J Integr Med 8:29–35

Santarelli RL, Pierre F, Corpet DE (2008) Processed meat and colorectal cancer: a review of epidemiologic and experimental evidence. Nutr Cancer 60:131–144

Smith S (2013) Mind-body intervention helps regulate stress hormone levels in nurses. EHS Today [Internet]. https://www.ehstoday.com/health/article/21918246/mindbody-intervention-helps-regulate-stress-hormone-levels-in-nurses

Takahara K, Sano K (2004) Life prolongation and QOL improvement effect of modified arabinoxylan from rice bran (BioBran/MGN-3) for progressive cancer. Clin Pharmacol Ther 14:267–271

Vickers AJ (2007) Which botanicals or other unconventional anticancer agents should we take to clinical trial? J Soc Integr Oncol 5:125–129

Volek J (2018) Ketogenic diet and chemotherapy in affecting recurrence in patients with stage iv breast cancer (keto-care) [Internet]. ClinicalTrials.gov. https://clinicaltrials.gov/ct2/show/NCT03535701

Wahbeh H, Haywood A, Kaufman K, Zwickey H (2009) Mind-body medicine and immune system outcomes: a systematic review. Open Complement Med J 1:25–34

Wikipedia (2020) Herbal medicine [Internet]. [cited 2020 Nov 30]. https://en.m.wikipedia.org/wiki/Herbalism

Witt CM, Balneaves LG, Cardoso MJ, Cohen L, Greenlee H, Johnstone P et al (2017) A comprehensive definition for integrative oncology. J Natl Cancer Inst Monogr 2017

Xu R (2019) Vitamin C intravenously with chemotherapy in advanced colorectal cancer [Internet]. ClinicalTrials.gov. [cited 2020 Nov 30]. https://clinicaltrials.gov/ct2/show/NCT02969681

Yamagiwa K, Ichikawa K (1918) Experimental study of the pathogenesis of carcinoma. J Cancer Res 3:1–29

The Therapeutic Application of RBAC in Cancer

6

Tibor Hajto

Abstract

Growing evidence suggests that the adaptive cytotoxic cells have prophylactic effects as they work more proficiently in the early phases of tumor development, whereas the innate cellular system acts more curatively in parallel with disease progression. However, both cellular systems depend on the balance of the innate immune system, in which the degree of pre-activation (priming) and polarity play an important role. Tumor-induced dysregulation of the innate immune system leads to decreased function of type 1 effector cells and a predominance of type 2 cells, promoting the development of tumors. Consequently, we must learn to manipulate this regulation by increasing the type 1 innate immune effector activity and diminishing the type 2 system. This balance can also play an important role in the sensitivity of tumor cells to innate effectors (such as natural killer cells), which are regulated by the expressions of stress-related receptors on tumor cells (such as MICA, MICB, or ULBP 1–3). Rice bran arabinoxylan compound (RBAC) has been shown to activate the type 1 effector cells given in doses of 10–45 mg/kg and, in a controlled clinical trial, was able to result in an evidence-based antitumor effect. Case reports suggest that a combination of RBAC with therapy modalities that increase the expression of stress-related molecules on tumor cells (using growth factor receptor inhibitors or lower doses of gemcitabine) can result in remarkable clinical results. Therefore, if we learn to better manipulate the immunoregulation using standardized RBAC together with appropriate oncological treatments, it may open new strategies in tumor therapy.

T. Hajto (✉)
Medical University Pecs, Törökbálint, Hungary
e-mail: drhajtot@t-online.hu

S. C. Pak et al. (eds.), *Modified Rice Bran Arabinoxylan*,
https://doi.org/10.1007/978-981-19-5735-2_6

Keywords

Biobran · Tumor development · Immune system · Oncology · NKG2D

6.1 Immunological Background

6.1.1 Tumor-Induced Immune Dysregulation

Despite the tremendous technical development of tumor diagnostics, at the time of the first recognition of malignant tumors with a higher diameter than 5 mm, the number of cancerous cells is in the millions. At this size, an outgrowth of clones that can definitively escape from T cell lysis is inevitable. It is also known that these T cell-resistant clones exhibit genetic dysregulation-related irreversible and unrepairable quantitative and qualitative alterations in their major histocompatibility complex (MHC)-I antigen production. Such alterations result in a growing inability to present tumor-associated antigens for the cytotoxic T cells (Seliger et al. 2000; Doan et al. 2008; Male et al. 2013). Therefore, growing attention is focusing on the MHC-I unrestricted innate immune mechanisms, whose escape mechanisms appear to be more reversible. It is well known that the MHC-I unrestricted effector cells have an essential priming activity that can determine their functions. Similar to the neuroendocrine system, this priming of the innate immune system also exhibits a polarity in that it is committed in two directions.

As shown in Fig. 6.1, the type 1 macrophages (M1) and monocytes which originated from type 1 dendritic cells (D1) generate proinflammatory cytokines for only a short time. They facilitate the production of interleukin (IL)-12 and activate cytotoxic effectors such as natural killer (NK), gamma/delta T, and type 1 NKT1 cells which are potent inhibitors of tumor growth in a MHC unrestricted manner (Sánchez-Torres et al. 2001; Mantovani 2007; Hajtó 2018). However, the type 1 innate immune cells are downregulated in tumor disease (Hajtó 2018). Moreover, available evidence suggests a tumor-induced dominance of type 2 macrophages (M2) and plasmacytoid precursors originated type 2 dendritic (D2) cells which produce IL-4 and IL-10. Together, they facilitate the generation of T helper (Th) 2 cells and inhibit the type 1 system (Mantovani 2007; Hajtó 2018; Murray 1998; Srivastava 2012). It was also shown that M2 and D2 cells affect chronic inflammation, promote cell proliferation by producing growth factors, and stimulate angiogenesis.

In parallel with the downregulation of type 1 cells, it was also found that tumor patients can have up to 40% type 2 upregulation of peripheral monocytes, which is in contrast to healthy persons who have only 10% (Sánchez-Torres et al. 2001; Mantovani 2007). In immunological research, there is further evidence that support this polarity. For example, in patients with pancreatic cancer, which has mostly a very unfavorable prognosis, the dominance of type 2 mechanisms appears to play a considerable role. It has been repeatedly shown that the peripheral level and cytotoxic activity of NK cells are positively correlated with cancer survival (Adamska

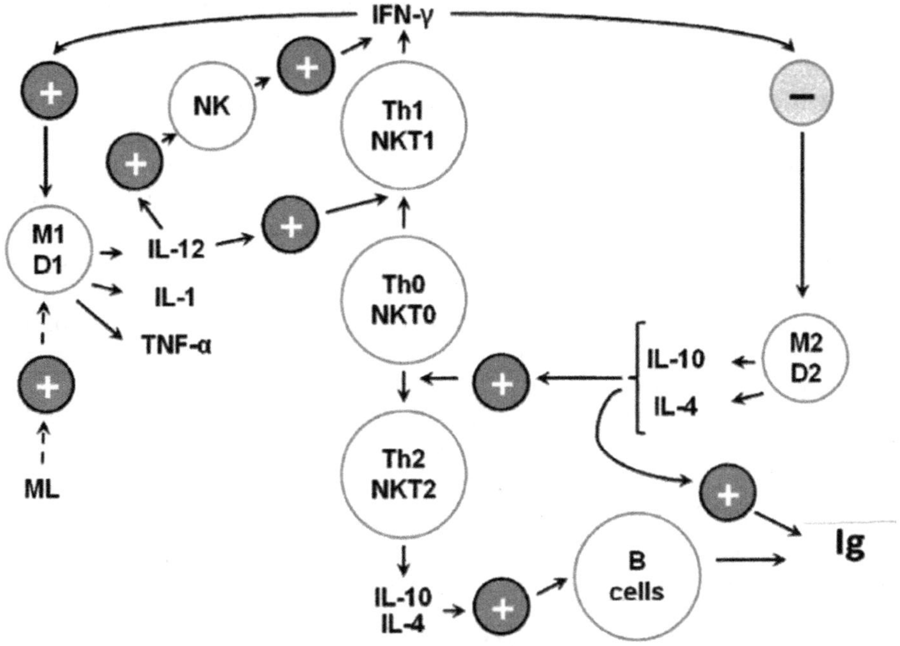

Fig. 6.1 The innate immune system is committed in two directions. M1 and D1 are type 1 macrophages and dendritic cells which take part in the regulation of the antitumor killer cells. M2 and D2 are type 2 macrophages and dendritic cells which facilitate the generation of Th2 cells and inhibit the type 1 system. (Adapted from Murray (Murray 1998))

et al. 2017; Davis et al. 2012). New evidence indicates that pancreatic carcinoma cells release metabolites favoring the expansion and accumulation of monocytic myeloid-derived suppressor cells, resulting in an increased level of both circulating and tumor-infiltrating type 2 innate immune cells. This imbalance between type 1 and type 2 mechanisms is associated with shorter overall survival of pancreatic carcinoma patients (Trovato et al. 2019).

Based on recent tumor immunological data, the immune surveillance theory has not been discarded (Srivastava 2012). This theory suggests that cancer cells frequently arise within the body, but they usually are eliminated before they multiply sufficiently. Most mutated cells never become cancer, and tumors arise only if they can escape immune surveillance. Consequently, it is assumed that adaptive T cells are more essential in prophylaxis than in healing.

6.1.2 Modulation of Innate Immune Mechanisms by RBAC

Over the past three decades, approximately 90% of tumor immunological research has focused on the adaptive T cells whose impaired function is described by their inadequate activation. However, this decades-long view is completely contradicted by the generally accepted opinion that tumors do not cause clinical signs of immune downregulation (e.g., frequent infections and altered immunological laboratory results, etc.). This opinion is further supported by clinical observations that certain malignancies are less common in acquired immunodeficiency syndrome (AIDS) patients (unpublished data). This is surprising since it is well known that AIDS patients show a collapse in the cellular adaptive immune system. However, it should be noted that during AIDS infection, the interaction between viral pathogen-associated molecular pattern (PAMP) molecules (such as gp120) and pattern recognition receptors (PRR) molecules on phagocytic cells in the host can upregulate the type 1 innate immune system, which is supported by several investigations (Capobianchi 1996; Kong et al. 1996). Could this AIDS-induced activation of the type 1 innate immune system result in an enhanced tumor defense? At present, this has not been investigated despite the fact that it would be apparent.

It is well known that the binding of PRR expressed on the phagocytic cell by appropriate PAMP molecules on pathogens can lead to the activation of the type 1 innate system causing an elevated MHC-I unrestricted host defense against tumor cells. In humans, PRR also includes toll-like receptors (TLR), mainly present on phagocytic cells and on a variety of other host cells, which recognize and bind to PAMP molecules to form interlocking structures and play a major role. As is well known, PRR/TLR agonists have had a long journey in the field of cancer immunotherapy (Bancroft 2012). Various bacteria have also been investigated to activate the type 1 natural immunity, but clinical success was inhibited mainly by the toxic side effects and tolerance. When the bacteria were killed, the structure of their PAMP molecules was also damaged.

Since PAMP molecules must be rigorously fitted to PRR, the biotechnology industry is encumbered to produce them. Although PAMP molecules can never exist in the host, they are widely found in nature. Consequently, growing attention is focusing on the PAMP-like molecules with plant origin, which have considerably fewer side effects in contrast to bacteria. At the moment, little research is available about PAMP-like plant immunomodulators. Unfortunately, the market is full of alternative but poorly investigated immunomodulators with scant evidence-based support.

The most investigated and evidence-based plant immunomodulator is an arabinoxylan extract from rice bran called rice bran arabinoxylan compound (RBAC) manufactured and supplied in a standardized form as BioBran/MGN-3 by Daiwa Pharmaceutical Co Ltd., Tokyo, Japan. It is composed of denatured hemicellulose, obtained by rice bran hemicellulose reacting with multiple carbohydrate hydrolyzing enzymes from shiitake mushrooms. RBAC preparations are standardized for their main chemical component: arabinoxylan with a xylose (in its main chain) and arabinose polymers (in its side chains). This plant immunomodulator strongly differs from other plant preparations since the enzymatic fermentation breaks down each glycolytic bond except for the binding between arabinose and xylose. This results in an arabinoxylan configuration with a similar form that exists in the plant and retains its PAMP-like properties. Indeed, this hydrolyzing enzyme-isolated RBAC has a similar immunomodulatory effect as

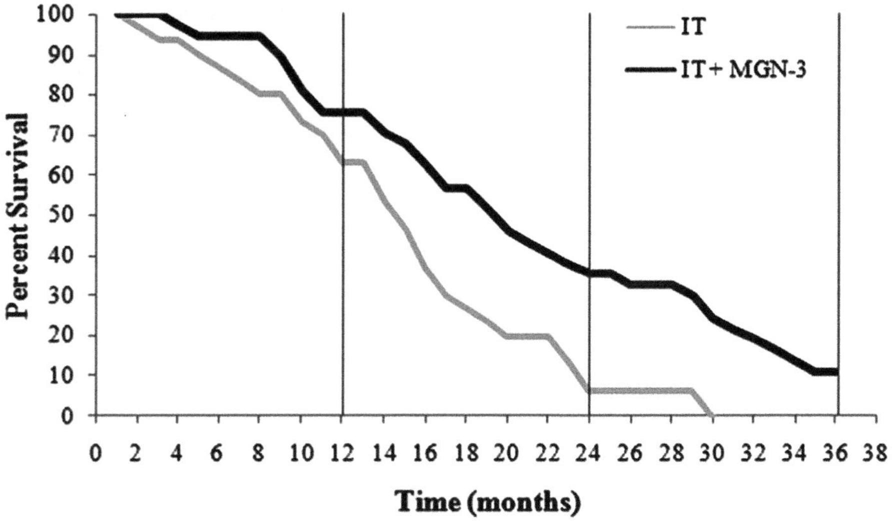

Fig. 6.2 In a 3-year randomized prospective, double-blind clinical trial, arabinoxylan concentrate (BioBran) was shown to enhance the effects of interventional chemotherapy against hepatocellular carcinoma. After 1 g Biobran daily for 12 months, the 2-year survival was 35% versus 6%. (Reproduced from Bang et al. (Bang et al. 2010))

bacterial PAMP molecules. A great number of publications report that a given dose between 15 and 45 mg/kg RBAC can activate the type 1 natural effectors, such as phagocytic and NK activities (Badr El-Din et al. 2008, 2016a, b; Pérez-Martínez et al. 2015; Tan and Norhaizan 2017; Cholujova et al. 2009, 2013; Ghoneum and Agrawal 2011, 2014; Ghoneum et al. 2013, 2014; Gollapudi and Ghoneum 2008), and exhibit clinical benefit (Bang et al. 2010; Itoh et al. 2015; McDermott et al. 2006).

As shown in Fig. 6.2, a double-blind, randomized clinical trial with liver cancer patients showed that RBAC given daily with a low dose for 12 months in parallel with chemotherapy was able to induce a six-fold increase in the 2-year survival rate (Bang et al. 2010). Despite the fact that RBAC is the most supported evidence-based and standardized plant immunomodulator without any side effects, it remains registered as a food supplement and not used in oncologic centers all over the world. Consequently, its clinical research is regularly hindered.

Human research ethics committees often refuse permission for cancer clinical trials with food supplements as interventions, and mainly case studies are allowed. The cautious behavior of ethics committees and oncologic centers with evidence-based food supplements is very regrettable since a possible manipulation of the polarity in the innate immune system could open up new perspectives in tumor research. Case reports always suggest more hypotheses that should be further investigated in clinical trials. Since the polarity of the neuroendocrine system with the polarity of the natural immune system exhibits a close relationship, a great number of preliminary clinical observations always become more exciting.

6.1.3 The Central Role of NKG2D as the Ligand for NK Cells

As discussed previously, the most important and most investigated MHC unrestricted killer cells are the NK cells, which have various receptors on their cell membrane. Among them is a tumor defense pivotal killer activator receptor, namely, the NKG2D. Their so-called stress-related ligands, such as MHC class I chain-related A and B (MICA/B) and UL-16 binding proteins (ULBP) 1–3, are widely expressed on various tumor cells. As was mentioned above, the loss of MHC-I antigens can decrease the sensitivity of tumor cells to T lymphocytes, but it can increase their sensitivity against NK and other MHC-I unrestricted killer cells (such as type 1 NKT or gamma/delta T cells). Parallel with the decrease in MHC-I expression, the upregulation of the stress-related ligands on tumor cells can enhance the effect of NK lysis which can further be increased by RBAC plant immunomodulator.

MICA and ULBP2 expression were found to be decreased with the progression of malignant tumors. A substantial number of studies show that the expression of stress molecules is influenced by various regulatory events (Martinez-Pomares 2012). For example, one of the most important regulatory substances (IL-4) in the type 2 innate system can selectively downregulate them. The dominance of M2 and D2 cells in tumor environment can lead to enhanced production of growth factors which can contribute not only to the downregulation of the type 1 natural effector cells but also to diminish the expression of the NKG2D ligands, resulting in a lower sensitivity of tumor targets to NK cells. Indeed, it was shown that epidermal growth factors can inhibit the NK cytotoxicity against cancer cells by downregulating the expression of ULBP 1–3 or MICA and MICB on the tumor cell membrane (Bae et al. 2012; He et al. 2013).

As mentioned, RBAC is the first standardized plant immunomodulator proven by a controlled and randomized clinical trial (Bang et al. 2010). If we stimulate the type 1 effector cells by RBAC and increase the sensitivity of tumor cells to them by growth factor receptor (GFR) inhibitors or gentamycin in parallel, then we can open new perspectives in tumor therapy with significant clinical results, which will be demonstrated later. Clinical investigations and case reports can also support that the regulation of both NKG2D and its stress-related ligands has crucial importance in tumor therapy.

6.2 Case Reports Which Support the Clinical Benefits of RBAC

6.2.1 A Patient with Lung Adenocarcinoma Treated with Erlotinib and RBAC

As mentioned, the stimulatory effect of GFR signaling pathway inhibitors on the expression of stress-related molecules results in enhanced sensitivity of tumor cells to NK cytotoxicity. Therefore, their combination with evidence-based immunomodulators is very promising. This is due to the potential increase in the

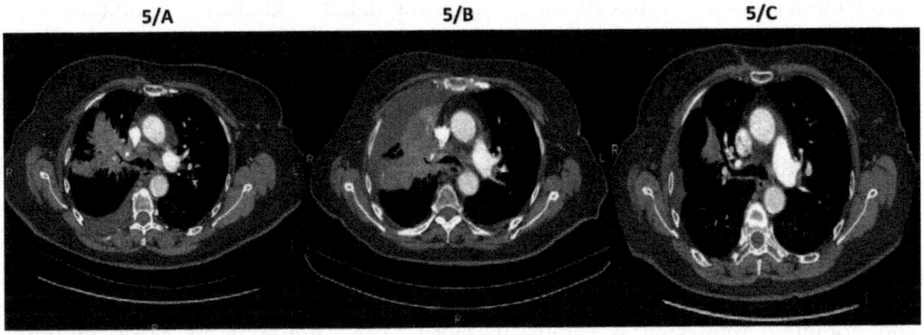

Fig. 6.3 Computerized tomography investigations of lungs in the patient with inoperable adenocarcinoma, which is localized on the boundary of the middle and lower right lobes which was accompanied with extensive atelectasis: 5/A, prior to the chemotherapy; 5/B, after four cycles of carboplatin (110 mg/m^2) and paclitaxel (90 mg/m^2); 5/C, 7 months after a combinative treatment with erlotinib (75 mg daily) and standardized plant immunomodulators giving 0.75 ng/kg VAA-I in extract and 45 mg/kg RBAC. (Reproduced from Hajtó (Hajtó et al. 2016))

NKG2D expression and thereby the cytotoxicity of NK cells against the tumor cells sensitized by GFR inhibitor. Indeed, the following case report may support this synergistic effect.

A 75-year-old patient with inoperable lung adenocarcinoma showed a very rapid progression during chemotherapy with four cycles of carboplatin and paclitaxel. The patient was in a terminal state. Therefore, the chemotherapy was stopped, and erlotinib (daily 75 mg Tarceva) was started in combination with RBAC treatment. As shown in Fig. 6.3, 7 months later, a computerized tomography (CT) scan established a nearly complete remission, and the duration of this remission was longer than 3 years (Hajtó et al. 2016).

Erlotinib belongs to the first agent to target tyrosine kinase of the epidermal GFR (EGFR). In clinical trials of patients with advanced non-small cell lung cancer (NSCLC) who had previously been treated with chemotherapy, the response rate to EGFR tyrosine kinase inhibitor was found to be between 8 and15% (Fukuoka et al. 2003; Shepherd et al. 2005). Interestingly, in a very large non-inferiority study, the median survivals of 1466 patients were compared after chemotherapy (75 mg/m^2 docetaxel every 3 weeks) versus EGFR inhibitor (250 mg/daily gefitinib), and no significant differences were found (Kim et al. 2008). Therefore, the potential synergistic effects of EGFR inhibitors with standardized RBAC can be promising.

6.2.2 A Patient with Carcinoma in the Biliary Duct Treated with Another GFR Signaling Pathway (MEK/BRAF) Inhibitor and RBAC

Similar to the combination with erlotinib, another exciting case report is shown with MEK/BRAF inhibitors combined with RBAC. As it is well known, MEK (mitogen-activated extracellular signal-regulated kinase) inhibitors can downregulate the MAPK (mitogen-activated protein kinase) cascade (RAS/RAF/MEK/ERK), which plays an important role in the enhanced cell cycle progression and migration in tumor patients. In the case of BRAF mutations, MEK and BRAF inhibitors have a synergistic effect. Similar to erlotinib, the MEK inhibitor can also upregulate the expression of stress-related molecules (MICA/B, ULBP1-3). In other words, the most significant effect of MEK/ERK signaling inhibitors is the recovery of tumor-induced decrease of NKG2D ligands (MICA/B and ULBP1-3) (Yang et al. 2017). However, despite their immune sensitivity enhancing effect, MEK inhibitors alone (without immunomodulator) can induce only a transient clinical remission, and complete remission is rarely observed. The outgrowth of MEK inhibitor-resistant clones within progressed tumors appears to be inevitable (Smith and Wellbrock 2016). Therefore, the astonishing results of the following case report, when MEK inhibitor was combined with high doses of RBAC, are encouraging.

A 58-year-old patient showed inoperable low differentiated adenocarcinoma in the biliary duct. After 30 GY irradiation and two cycles of chemotherapy (gemcitabine and cisplatin), she had a very rapid progression of lung, liver, and brain metastases as revealed by CT and magnetic resonance (MR) investigations. The patient was nearly terminal. The chemotherapy was stopped, and treatment with MEK and BRAF inhibitors was started in combination with daily 45 mg/kg RBAC. After 4 weeks, a rapid improvement of her disease was observed. Eight months later, near complete remissions of all metastases were established by CT and MR (Hajtó 2017). Figure 6.4 demonstrates the complete remission of brain metastasis in the cerebellum and the rapid improvement of her tumor marker.

The positive results of these two case reports (Hajtó et al. 2016; Hajtó 2017) can suggest the hypothesis that the enhancing effect on NKG2D expression by RBAC in parallel with the upregulating expression of stress-related ligands by GFR signaling pathway inhibitors may result in a synergistic clinical benefit. Further clinical investigations are necessary to prove this hypothesis, but we need more acceptance for evidence-based immunomodulators for this aim.

6.2.3 Effect of Cytostatic Therapy on the Stress-Related NKG2D Ligands on Tumor Cells

Clinical observations can often suggest a clinical benefit if conventional cytostatic treatment is combined with RBAC. For example, Bang et al. found through a double-blind clinical trial that the 2-year survival rate for liver cancer patients treated with RBAC together with conventional chemotherapy was six-fold higher than those without RBAC (Bang et al. 2010). Consequently, the question arose as to whether several cytostatic drugs can also enhance the expression of NKG2D ligands resulting in enhanced sensitivity to MHC-I unrestricted killer mechanisms. At present, insufficient data is available. However, the interesting results of Morisaki et al. (Morisaki et al. 2014) must be mentioned. These authors investigated the effect of gemcitabine on MICA/B expression in the culture of T24 urothelial cancer cells. At a dose of

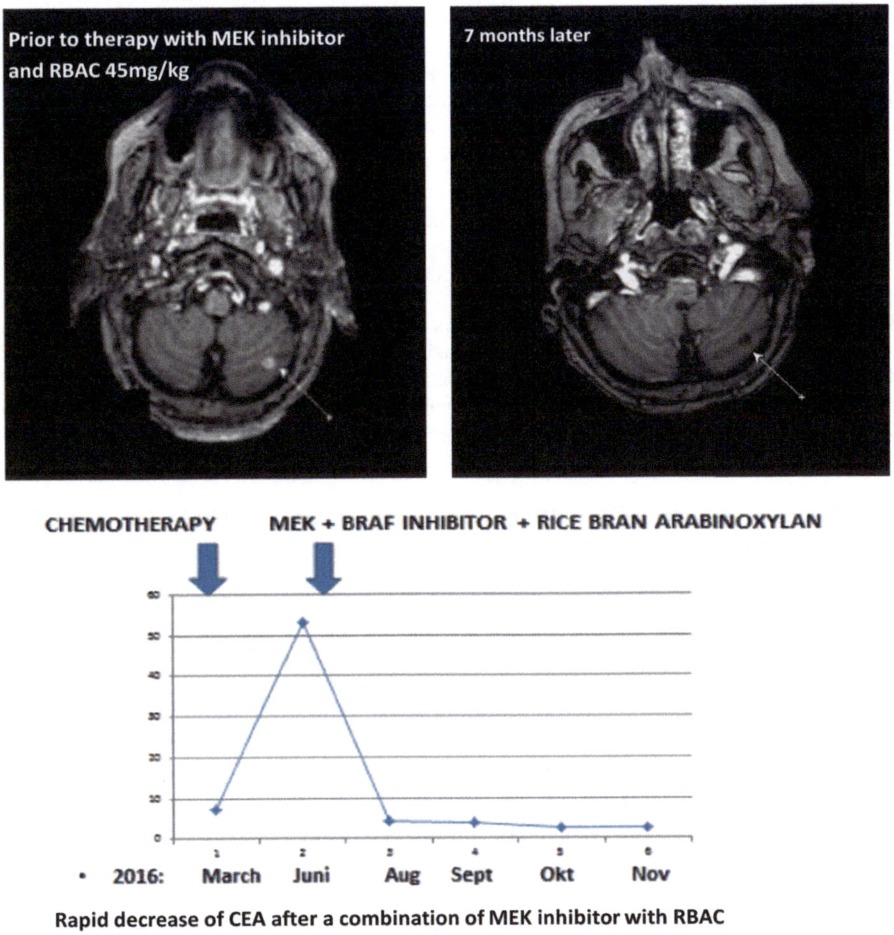

Fig. 6.4 Magnetic resonance (MR) investigations of a patient with biliary duct cancer represent a complete remission after treatment with 1 × 2 mg trametinib and 2 × 150 mg dabrafenib combined with 45 mg rice bran arabinoxylan concentrate. In parallel to the MR investigation, the level of carcinoembryonic antigen (CEA) also showed a rapid normalization as displayed in the bottom graph. (Reproduced from Hajtó (Hajtó 2017))

0.1 μg/ml, gemcitabine induced more than twice the increase in expression of MICA/B on cancer cells. Interestingly, higher doses (e.g., 1 μg/ml) were less effective. Other authors have also established similar results (Okita et al. 2015; Xie et al. 2017). It was also shown that the NK sensitivity of T24 urothelial cancer cells in the presence of gemcitabine with and without IL-2 was also elevated (Morisaki et al. 2014). Clinical case reports can further support these in vitro results.

In January 2020, a 56-year-old patient showed in the caudal part of the pancreas an inoperable ductal adenocarcinoma (39 × 46 mm) with multiplex liver metastases (10–30 mm), as established by CT and biopsy. His tumor markers were elevated:

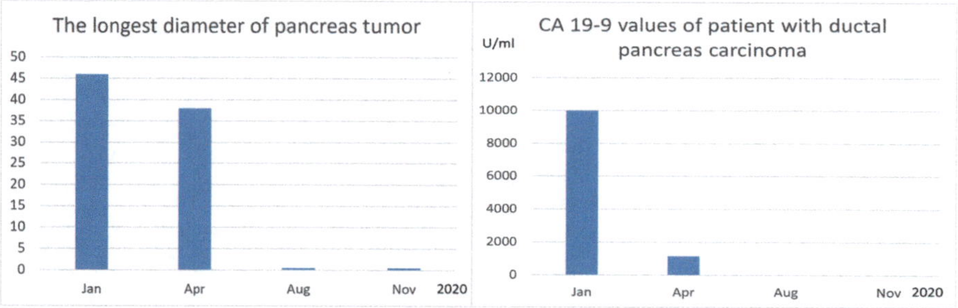

Fig. 6.5 Monitoring the greatest tumor diameters and the tumor markers (CA 19–9) of a patient with inoperable pancreatic ductal adenocarcinoma. Largest tumor diameters and CA 19–9 values of the patient with metastatic pancreatic ductal adenocarcinoma after treatment for 10 months with eight cycles of gemcitabine and nab-paclitaxel combined with standardized rice bran arabinoxylan concentrate (MGN-3/Biobran)

carbohydrate antigen (CA) 19-9 was higher than 10,000 U/ml, and the carcinoembryonic antigen (CEA) level was 26.76 ng/ml. He was nearly terminal (having a 27 kg decrease in body weight and intensive pains). From February 2020 until August 2021, he was treated with 800 mg/m^2 gemcitabine on the first, eighth, and fifteenth days every month. The first gemcitabine treatments were combined with nab-paclitaxel. From February 2020, the chemotherapy was regularly combined with 45 mg/kg RBAC given per os three times a week (Monday, Tuesday, and Friday). In April 2020, a remission of pancreas tumor (25 × 38 mm) and an average 3–10 mm decrease in liver metastases were established by CT. Tumor markers were also decreased: CA 19-9 was 1172 U/ml and CEA 3.0 ng/ml. In August 2020, complete remission of the pancreatic tumor was found, and the liver metastases showed further 3–6 mm decreases. The tumor markers were normalized (CA 19-9 was 22 U/ml and CEA was 2.0 ng/ml).

Figure 6.5 demonstrates the results of monitoring the tumor diameters and the CA 19-9 level. In November 2020, the complete remission of the pancreatic tumor was reported with a CA 19-9 level of 14.5 U/ml. In addition, the liver metastases showed complete remissions. The patient, after treatment for 10 months, had no complaints and could return to work. This complete remission with normal tumor markers and excellent quality of life in August 2021 (after the start of therapy for 18 months) was also established.

6.3 Conclusion

RBAC belongs to the most investigated, standardized, and evidence-based plant immunomodulators, which can improve the tumor-induced dysregulation of the innate immune system. RBAC has been shown to increase the survival of patients with advanced tumor disease in a controlled clinical trial and among case reports.

The clinical research of RBAC can also support the NKG2D receptors on NK cells and their stress-related ligands on tumor cells which are pivotal regulator molecules in the tumor defense. Case reports also suggest the hypothesis that activation of NKG2D by RBAC in combination with the stimulation of expression of their ligands (MICA/B and ULBP1-3) by GFR inhibitors or with lower doses of gemcitabine may open innovative approaches in tumor therapy.

References

Adamska A, Domenichini A, Falasca M (2017) Pancreatic ductal adenocarcinoma: current and evolving therapies. Int J Mol Sci 18:1338

Badr El-Din NK, Noaman E, Ghoneum M (2008) In vivo tumor inhibitory effects of nutritional rice bran supplement MGN-3/Biobran on ehrlich carcinoma-bearing mice. Nutr Cancer 60:235–244

Badr El-Din NK, Ali DA, Alaa El-Dein M, Ghoneum M (2016a) Enhancing the apoptotic effect of a low dose of paclitaxel on tumor cells in mice by arabinoxylan rice bran (MGN-3/Biobran). Nutr Cancer 68:1010–1020

Badr El-Din NK, Abdel Fattah SM, Pan D, Tolentino L, Ghoneum M (2016b) Chemopreventive activity of MGN-3/Biobran against chemical induction of glandular stomach carcinogenesis in rats and its apoptotic effect in gastric cancer cells. Integr Cancer Ther 15:NP26. https://doi.org/10.1177/1534735416642287

Bae J-H, Kim S-J, Kim M-J, Oh S-O, Chung J-S, Kim S-H, Kang C-D (2012) Susceptibility to natural killer cell-mediated lysis of colon cancer cells is enhanced by treatment with epidermal growth factor receptor inhibitors through UL16-binding protein-1 induction. Cancer Sci 103:7–16

Bancroft GJ (2012) Immunity to bacteria and fungi. In: Male D, Brostoff J, Roth D, Roitt I (eds) Immunology, 8th edn. Elsevier, London / Philadelphia, pp 223–242

Bang MH, Van Riep T, Thinh NT et al (2010) Arabinoxylan rice bran (MGN-3) enhances the effects of interventional therapies for the treatment of hepatocellular carcinoma: a three-year randomized clinical trial. Anticancer Res 30:5145–5151

Capobianchi MR (1996) Induction of lymphomonocyte activation by HIV-1 glycoprotein gp120. Possible role in AIDS pathogenesis. J Biol Regul Homeost Agents 10:83–91

Cholujova D, Jakubikova J, Sedlak J (2009) BioBran-augmented maturation of human monocyte-derived dendritic cells. Neoplasma 56:89–95

Cholujova D, Jakubikova J, Czako B, Martisova M, Hunakova L, Duraj J, Mistrik M, Sedlak J (2013) MGN-3 arabinoxylan rice bran modulates innate immunity in multiple myeloma patients. Cancer Immunol Immunother 62:437–445

Davis M, Conlon K, Bohac GC, Barcenas J, Leslie W, Watkins L, Lamzabi I, Deng Y, Li Y, Plate JMD (2012) Effect of pemetrexed on innate immune killer cells and adaptive immune T cells in subjects with adenocarcinoma of the pancreas. J Immunother 35:629–640

Doan T, Melvold R, Viselli S, Waltenbaugh C (2008) Presentation by MHC class I. In: Harvey RA, Champe PC (eds) Immunology, 1st edn. Lippincott Williams and Wilkins, Philadelphia, PA, pp 123–126

Fukuoka M, Yano S, Giaccone G et al (2003) Multi-institutional randomized phase II trial of gefitinib for previously treated patients with advanced non-small-cell lung cancer (the IDEAL 1 trial) [corrected]. J Clin Oncol 21:2237–2246

Ghoneum M, Agrawal S (2011) Activation of human monocyte-derived dendritic cells in vitro by the biological response modifier arabinoxylan rice bran (MGN-3/Biobran). Int J Immunopathol Pharmacol 24:941–948

Ghoneum M, Agrawal S (2014) MGN-3/Biobran enhances generation of cytotoxic CD8+ T cells via upregulation of DEC-205 expression on dendritic cells. Int J Immunopathol Pharmacol 27: 523–530

Ghoneum M, Badr El-Din NK, Fattah SMA, Tolentino L (2013) Arabinoxylan rice bran (MGN-3/Biobran) provides protection against whole-body γ-irradiation in mice via restoration of hematopoietic tissues. J Radiat Res 54:419

Ghoneum M, Badr El-Din NK, Ali DA, El-Dein MA (2014) Modified arabinoxylan from rice bran, MGN-3/Biobran, sensitizes metastatic breast cancer cells to paclitaxel in vitro. Anticancer Res 34:81–87

Gollapudi S, Ghoneum M (2008) MGN-3/Biobran, modified arabinoxylan from rice bran, sensitizes human breast cancer cells to chemotherapeutic agent, daunorubicin. Cancer Detect Prev 32:1–6

Hajtó T (2017) Can a standardized plant immunomodulator (rice bran arabinoxylan concentrate/MGN-3) increase the effects of MEK and BRAF inhibitors with clinical benefit? Case report of a patient with carcinoma in biliary duct. Res Rev Insights 1:1–4

Hajtó T (2018) New perspectives to improve the MHC-I unrestricted immune mechanisms against malignant tumors. Adv Clin Transl Res 2:100015

Hajtó T, Horváth A, Baranyai L, Kuzma M, Perjési P (2016) Can the EGFR inhibitors increase the immunomodulatory effects of standardized plant extracts (mistletoe lectin and arabinoxylan) with clinical benefit? Case report of a patient with lung adenocarcinoma. Clin Case Reports Rev 2:456–459

He S, Yin T, Li D et al (2013) Enhanced interaction between natural killer cells and lung cancer cells: involvement in gefitinib-mediated immunoregulation. J Transl Med 11:186

Itoh Y, Mizuno M, Ikeda M, Nakahara R, Kubota S, Ito J, Okada T, Kawamura M, Kikkawa F, Naganawa S (2015) A randomized, double-blind pilot trial of hydrolyzed rice bran versus placebo for radioprotective effect on acute gastroenteritis secondary to chemoradiotherapy in patients with cervical cancer. Evid Based Complement Alternat Med 2015:974390

Kim ES, Hirsh V, Mok T et al (2008) Gefitinib versus docetaxel in previously treated non-small-cell lung cancer (INTEREST): a randomised phase III trial. Lancet 372:1809–1818

Kong LY, Wilson BC, McMillian MK, Bing G, Hudson PM, Hong JS (1996) The effects of the HIV-1 envelope protein gp120 on the production of nitric oxide and proinflammatory cytokines in mixed glial cell cultures. Cell Immunol 172:77–83

Male D, Brostoff J, Roth DB, Roitt I (2013) Immunity to cancer. In: Hyde M, Vosburgh A (eds) Immunology. Elsevier, pp 355–365

Mantovani A (2007) Inflammation and cancer: the macrophage connection. Medicina (B Aires) 67: 32–34

Martinez-Pomares L (2012) Mononuclear phagocytes in immune defense. In: Male D, Brostoff J, Roth D, Roitt I (eds) Immunology, 8th edn. Elsevier, London, pp 125–142

McDermott C, Richards SCM, Thomas PW, Montgomery J, Lewith G (2006) A placebo-controlled, double-blind, randomized controlled trial of a natural killer cell stimulant (BioBran MGN-3) in chronic fatigue syndrome. QJM 99:461–468

Morisaki T, Hirano T, Koya N, Kiyota A, Tanaka H, Umebayashi M, Onishi H, Katano M (2014) NKG2D-directed cytokine-activated killer lymphocyte therapy combined with gemcitabine for patients with chemoresistant metastatic solid tumors. Anticancer Res 34:4529–4538

Murray JS (1998) How the MHC selects Th1/Th2 immunity. Immunol Today 19:157–163

Okita R, Wolf D, Yasuda K et al (2015) Contrasting effects of the cytotoxic anticancer drug gemcitabine and the EGFR tyrosine kinase inhibitor gefitinib on NK cell-mediated cytotoxicity via regulation of NKG2D ligand in non-small-cell lung cancer cells. PLoS One 10:e0139809

Pérez-Martínez A, Valentín J, Fernández L et al (2015) Arabinoxylan rice bran (MGN-3/Biobran) enhances natural killer cell-mediated cytotoxicity against neuroblastoma in vitro and in vivo. Cytotherapy 17:601–612

Sánchez-Torres C, García-Romo GS, Cornejo-Cortés MA, Rivas-Carvalho A, Sánchez-Schmitz G (2001) CD16+ and CD16− human blood monocyte subsets differentiate in vitro to dendritic cells with different abilities to stimulate CD4+ T cells. Int Immunol 13:1571–1581

Seliger B, Maeurer MJ, Ferrone S (2000) Antigen-processing machinery breakdown and tumor growth. Immunol Today 21:455–464

Shepherd FA, Rodrigues Pereira J, Ciuleanu T et al (2005) Erlotinib in previously treated non-small-cell lung cancer. N Engl J Med 353:123–132

Smith MP, Wellbrock C (2016) Molecular pathways: maintaining MAPK inhibitor sensitivity by targeting nonmutational tolerance. Clin Cancer Res 22:5966–5970

Srivastava PK (2012) Immunity of cancer. In: Male D, Brostoff J, Roth D, Roitt I (eds) Immunology, 8th edn. Elsevier, London, pp 355–368

Tan BL, Norhaizan ME (2017) Scientific evidence of rice by-products for cancer prevention: chemopreventive properties of waste products from rice milling on carcinogenesis in vitro and in vivo. Biomed Res Int 2017:1–18

Trovato R, Fiore A, Sartori S et al (2019) Immunosuppression by monocytic myeloid-derived suppressor cells in patients with pancreatic ductal carcinoma is orchestrated by STAT3. J Immunother Cancer 7:255

Xie X, Zhou Y, Wang X, Guo J, Li J, Fan H, Dou J, Shen B, Zhou C (2017) Enhanced antitumor activity of gemcitabine by polysaccharide-induced NK cell activation and immune cytotoxicity reduction in vitro/vivo. Carbohydr Polym 173:360–371

Yang L, Shen M, Xu LJ, Yang X, Tsai Y, Keng PC, Chen Y, Lee SO (2017) Enhancing NK cell-mediated cytotoxicity to cisplatin-resistant lung cancer cells via MEK/Erk signaling inhibition. Sci Rep 7:7958

Radiation Therapy

7

Jerickson Abbie S. Flores and Jaffar C. Pineda

Abstract

Radiotherapy is an established modality in cancer treatment alone or in combination with other modalities such as surgery and chemotherapy. Although radiotherapy is employed to improve the quality of life (QoL), its association with several side effects remains a clinical challenge. Several studies have shown that treatment-related symptoms and side effects increased in general during radiotherapy due to inflammation and cytotoxic damage, eventually leading to unnecessary treatment interruptions or delays. Studies have shown that prolonged radiotherapy treatment time is associated with worse overall survival and poor quality of life among cancer patients undergoing treatment. This chapter explores the benefits of using rice bran arabinoxylan (Biobran) as a supportive treatment for cancer patients undergoing radiotherapy. This chapter also aims to analyze its impact on clinical outcomes based on several factors, including, but not limited to, hematologic parameters, nutritional status, treatment-related toxicities, and QoL. As of writing, only a few articles have been published on rice bran arabinoxylan's effects on cancer patients undergoing radiotherapy.

Keywords

Radiotherapy · Cancer treatment · Rice bran arabinoxylan · Biobran

J. A. S. Flores (✉) · J. C. Pineda
Department of Radiotherapy, Jose R. Reyes Memorial Medical Center, Manila, Philippines

S. C. Pak et al. (eds.), *Modified Rice Bran Arabinoxylan*,
https://doi.org/10.1007/978-981-19-5735-2_7

7.1 Introduction

Radiotherapy is an established modality in managing many malignancies either as definitive, neoadjuvant, or adjuvant treatment (Halperin et al. 2019). Although radiotherapy is employed to improve life quality, its association with several side effects remains a clinical limitation (Bese et al. 2007). Several studies have shown that treatment-related symptoms and side effects increased in general during radiotherapy due to inflammation and cytotoxic damage, which eventually leads to unnecessary treatment interruptions or delays (Astrup et al. 2017). The unnecessary adverse events of treatment will also affect the oncologic outcomes of cancer treatment. The body of literature has shown that prolonged radiotherapy treatment time is associated with worse overall survival among cancer patients undergoing treatment (Shaikh et al. 2016). Many clinical trials reported that the quality of life (QoL) of cancer patients was greatly affected during radiotherapy due to its treatment-associated side effects (Astrup et al. 2017). This chapter explores the benefits of using rice bran arabinoxylan (Biobran) as a supportive treatment for cancer patients undergoing radiotherapy. This chapter also aims to analyze its impact on clinical outcomes based on several factors such as, but not limited to, hematologic parameters, nutritional status, treatment-related toxicities, and QoL. As of writing, only a few articles have been published on rice bran arabinoxylan's effects among cancer patients undergoing radiotherapy.

7.2 Biological Effects of Rice Bran Arabinoxylan and Radiation Therapy

Radiation therapy's main biological effect is a consequence of the deoxyribonucleic acid (DNA) damage as the critical target. This action of radiation can be either direct or indirect. The direct action of radiation results from the interaction with the critical target in the cell DNA, either by excitation or ionization, which eventually leads to biological damage. In contrast, with indirect action, radiation interacts with other atoms or molecules such as water (comprising 80 percent of cellular composition) to produce free radicals, eventually causing oxidative damage to the critical target DNA. The indirect action of radiation can be modified by different factors, grouped as either radioprotectors or radiosensitizers. Radiation can affect both the tumor cells and the nearby normal cells resulting in clinical tumoricidal activity and side effects. Thus, the treatment goal is to achieve good oncologic outcomes (local control, disease-free survival, and overall survival) while minimizing treatment-related side effects (Hall and Giaccia 2019).

Rice bran arabinoxylan, also known as Biobran, is a natural blend of hemicellulose product of rice bran that is partially hydrolyzed using shiitake mushroom enzymes (*Lentinus edodes* mycelia extract), wherein the principal ingredient is the arabinoxylan compound or β-1, 4 xylophyronase hemicellulose (Maeda 2003). The immunomodulatory property and antitumor activity have been attributed to its complex heteropolysaccharide structure (arabinogalactan, arabinoxylan, arabinan, β-1,3:1,4-glucan) (Miura et al. 2013). Biobran is also attributed biologically to its radioprotective mechanism through its anti-oxidative properties that minimize radiation-related side effects while not affecting treatment effectivity and success (Ghoneum et al. 2013).

7.3 Animal Studies on Rice Bran Arabinoxylan and Radiation Therapy

Several animal studies have shown the beneficial effects of using Biobran with radiation therapy. Ghoneum et al. (2013) examined the radioprotective effects of Biobran on hematopoietic tissue after γ-irradiation in mice. Biobran pre-treatment resulted in the protection of hematologic parameters, specifically in bone marrow cellularity changes against irradiation-induced damage. It also showed splenic protection with Biobran. The study demonstrated the anti-oxidative activity in whole-body irradiated mice and attributed this to the protection from radiation-induced loss of body and organ weight. The study concluded that Biobran has the potential to have radioprotective effects on bone marrow progenitor cells, which suggests the possible use of Biobran as a supportive treatment to minimize the severe radiation-induced side effects.

Another study by Badr El-Din et al. (2019) opens the possibility of Biobran for enhancing radiation treatment efficacy. The radiosensitizing/radioenhancing effects were attributed to the observed enhanced induction of tumor cell apoptosis while conserving body and organ weight and maintaining normal liver enzyme levels. These results suggest that Biobran may be used to enhance the therapeutic effect of ionizing radiation in the treatment of solid tumors while minimizing its side effects on normal cells.

In a study by Zhao et al. (2020), Biobran was shown to be an excellent antioxidant and radioprotector. The study demonstrated that it could effectively protect mice against radiation-induced intestinal barrier dysfunction. These results suggest that Biobran can alleviate radiation-induced intestinal injury.

These animal studies show the possibilities of exploring the mechanism of Biobran as an adjunct to radiotherapy. However, future biological studies are needed to further explore the exact mechanism of Biobran at the molecular level, as both a radiosensitizer/radioenhancer to promote tumor cell killing and a potent radioprotector to minimize unwanted treatment-related side effects to the normal tissues.

7.4 Clinical Studies on Rice Bran Arabinoxylan and Radiation Therapy

Currently, only a few articles have been published on Biobran's effects among cancer patients undergoing radiotherapy.

In a study on patient clinical experiences by Tsunekawa (2004), among 16 progressive cancer patients who underwent conventional treatments including surgery, chemotherapy, and radiotherapy, long-term Biobran administration as immunomodulating nutritional support was shown to be safe and with no adverse effects, as noted among patients. Furthermore, the count of leukocyte, neutrophil, and lymphocyte as well as natural killer cell activity was reported to normalize if not improved after Biobran administration. A placebo-controlled, double-blind study published in 2015 by Itoh et al. (2015) on women with cervical cancer undergoing chemoradiotherapy showed lower diarrheal side effect assessment scores with the administration of Biobran. The study results suggest the possible radioprotective effects of Biobran on acute gastroenteritis among cervical cancer patients undergoing concurrent chemoradiotherapy (Itoh et al. 2015). In a study by Hajtó et al. (2016), 35 cancer patients (mostly advanced at stage II to IV) were given immunomodulating treatment, including mistletoe lectin and Biobran, for at least 6 months together with standard oncologic therapy. QoL questionnaires were completed, and the results showed some benefits in QoL scores, with the most important findings being the improvement of physical activity (71%) and appetite (66%). The study gives a special focus on the possible role of immunological processes in the impaired QoL of cancer patients. It suggests possible synergistic effects of Biobran and mistletoe lectin on immunomodulation, specifically natural killer cells and phagocytic activities (Hajtó et al. 2016).

An evidence-based review on Biobran as a complementary therapy for conventional cancer treatment was published in 2018 (Ooi et al. 2018). The study primarily aims to comprehensively review the available evidence on the effects and efficacies of Biobran as a complementary therapy for conventional cancer treatment. According to the analysis, previous clinical trials have shown that Biobran has promising effects as an adjunct therapy during conventional cancer treatment, which includes radiotherapy. The benefits include immunomodulatory effects, reduced treatment-related side effects (diarrhea, anorexia, nausea, vomiting, and others), improved QoL, and better oncologic treatment outcomes. Although the outcome improvement and reduction of treatment side effects are attributed to the immunomodulating activity of Biobran as proposed and mentioned in the previous animal and clinical studies, more research is needed to explore Biobran as a complementary treatment to conventional cancer therapy (Ooi et al. 2018).

In the latest study (Tan and Flores 2020) by a team of radiation oncologists, 65 head and neck cancer patients undergoing radiochemotherapy were enrolled in a randomized, double-blind clinical trial and were given either Biobran or placebo. The results showed that upon completion of radiochemotherapy, patients treated with Biobran showed significantly higher mean hematologic parameters, including hemoglobin, hematocrit, RBC, and platelets with significantly higher neutrophil and lymphocyte count. The Biobran arm also showed significantly better QoL and lower treatment-related toxicities compared to the placebo group. A subgroup analysis in the study also showed that patients given Biobran had lower rates of blood transfusion and hospital admission and no incidence of tumor progression, infection, and metastases compared to placebo. These have led to lesser treatment delays, avoidance of treatment mortalities and morbidities, more patients completing the treatment, and improved QoL among head and neck cancer patients undergoing radiochemotherapy. This study suggests that Biobran can be a potential adjunct in preventing radiation-induced side effects among head and neck cancer patients (Tan and Flores 2020).

7.5 Future Directions

Previous clinical studies and systematic reviews have shown that Biobran beneficially affects hematologic parameters, nutritional status, treatment-related toxicities, QoL, and oncologic outcomes. Although promising results are presented in these articles and studies, further research is needed to explore other potential effects and efficacy of Biobran as an adjunct treatment with conventional cancer therapy such as radiotherapy. More randomized controlled clinical trials with longer treatment follow-ups (5–10 years ideally) and other cancer-specific types are needed to further explore the benefits of Biobran as a supportive and complementary treatment for cancer patients undergoing radiotherapy with or without other conventional cancer therapies.

References

Astrup GL, Rustøen T, Hofsø K, Gran JM, Bjordal K (2017) Symptom burden and patient characteristics: association with quality of life in patients with head and neck cancer undergoing radiotherapy. Head Neck 39:2114–2126

Badr El-Din NK, Areida SK, Ahmed KO, Ghoneum M (2019) Arabinoxylan rice bran (MGN-3/ Biobran) enhances radiotherapy in animals bearing Ehrlich ascites carcinoma. J Radiat Res 60: 747–758

Bese NS, Hendry J, Jeremic B (2007) Effects of prolongation of overall treatment time due to unplanned interruptions during radiotherapy of different tumor sites and practical methods for compensation. Int J Radiat Oncol Biol Phys 68:654–661

Ghoneum M, Badr El-Din NK, Fattah SMA, Tolentino L (2013) Arabinoxylan rice bran (MGN-3/ Biobran) provides protection against whole-body γ-irradiation in mice via restoration of hematopoietic tissues. J Radiat Res 54:419

Hajtó T, Horvath A, Papp S (2016) Improvement of quality of life in tumor patients after an immunomodulatory treatment with standardized mistletoe lectin and arabinoxylan plant extracts. Int J Neurorehabil 3:2–4

Hall EJ, Giaccia AJ (2019) Radiobiology for the radiologist, 8th edn. Wolters Kluwer, Philadelphia, PA

Halperin EC, Wazer DE, Perez CA, Brady LW (2019) The discipline of radiation oncology. In: Halperin EC, Wazer DE, Perez CA, Brady LW (eds) Perez & Brady's principles and practice of radiation oncology, 7th edn. Wolters Kluwer, Philadelphia, PA, pp 94–96

Itoh Y, Mizuno M, Ikeda M, Nakahara R, Kubota S, Ito J et al (2015) A randomized, double-blind pilot trial of hydrolyzed rice bran versus placebo for radioprotective effect on acute gastroenteritis secondary to chemoradiotherapy in patients with cervical cancer. Evid Based Complement Alternat Med 2015:974390

Maeda H (2003) Scientific studies on the effectiveness and mechanism of Biobran MGN-3 [Internet]. [cited 2020 Nov 25]. https://www.biobran.org/overview#overview-for-practitioners

Miura T, Chiba M, Miyazaki Y, Kato Y, Maeda H (2013) Chemical structure of the component involved in immunoregulation. BioBran/MGN-3 (Rice bran Arab compound) Basic Clin Appl to Integr Med, 2nd edn. BioBran Research Foundation, Tokyo, pp 14–22

Ooi SL, McMullen D, Golombick T, Pak SC (2018) Evidence-based review of BioBran/MGN-3 arabinoxylan compound as a complementary therapy for conventional cancer treatment. Integr Cancer Ther 17:165–178

Shaikh T, Handorf EA, Murphy CT, Mehra R, Ridge JA, Galloway TJ (2016) The impact of radiation treatment time on survival in patients with head and neck cancer. Int J Radiat Oncol Biol Phys 96:967–975

Tan DFS, Flores JAS (2020) The immunomodulating effects of arabinoxylan rice bran (Lentin) on hematologic profile, nutritional status and quality of life among head and neck carcinoma patients undergoing radiation therapy: a double blind randomized control trial. Radiol J 12: 11–16

Tsunekawa H (2004) Effect of long-term administration of immunomodulatory food on cancer patients completing conventional treatments. Clin Pharmacol Ther 14:295–302

Zhao Z, Cheng W, Qu W, Wang K (2020) Arabinoxylan rice bran (MGN-3/Biobran) alleviates radiation-induced intestinal barrier dysfunction of mice in a mitochondrion-dependent manner. Biomed Pharmacother 124:109855

Health-Related Quality of Life

8

Soo Liang Ooi, Sok Cheon Pak, and Peter S. Micalos

Abstract

Being diagnosed with cancer is an emotionally traumatic event that adversely affects a patient's sense of overall function and wellbeing. Inflammation is a hallmark of cancer, with the inflammatory process aiding the proliferation and survival of malignant cells, suppressing the adaptive immune response while promoting tumour metastasis. Research has shown that rising systemic inflammation inversely correlates with the patients' reported quality of life (QoL) and is a vital underlying mechanism leading to poor prognostic outcomes in advanced cancer. Chronic inflammation alongside cancer treatment regimens also contributes to microglial activation in the central nervous system, causing neuroinflammation. This leads to behavioural comorbidities such as depression, anxiety, fatigue, cognitive impairment, and neuropathic pain, which also adversely affect the QoL. Cancer-related malnutrition due to the activation of systemic inflammation is also a predictive factor for poor QoL. Hence, targeting inflammation is a promising approach to enhancing cancer patients' QoL and improving treatment outcomes. Rice bran arabinoxylan compound (RBAC) is used among cancer patients to support weakened immune function during and after conventional cancer treatment. RBAC has been shown to be a safe and effective plant-based biological response modifier with immunomodulating and anti-inflammatory properties that can improve QoL. RBAC modulates the immune and inflammatory responses via direct absorption into the bloodstream and indirect modulation of gut microbiota. Numerous case studies and clinical trials have demonstrated improved QoL using RBAC among cancer patients.

S. L. Ooi · S. C. Pak (✉) · P. S. Micalos
School of Dentistry and Medical Sciences, Charles Sturt University, Bathurst, NSW, Australia
e-mail: spak@csu.edu.au

S. C. Pak et al. (eds.), *Modified Rice Bran Arabinoxylan*,
https://doi.org/10.1007/978-981-19-5735-2_8

However, further research is required to substantiate the effect of RBAC on the QoL of cancer patients using validated instruments.

Keywords

Biobran · Immunomodulator · Inflammation · Behavioural comorbidities · QLQ-C30 · FACT-G

8.1 Quality of Life of Cancer Patients

The World Health Organization defines quality of life (QoL) as "an individual's perception of their position in life in the context of the culture and value systems in which they live and in relation to their goals, expectations, standards and concerns" (World Health Organization 2021). Health-related QoL thus refers to how disease and treatment affects an individual's sense of overall function and wellbeing. The diagnosis of cancer is an emotionally traumatic event that instantly affects QoL. A patient's QoL changes as the disease progresses over time. Patients with nonmetastatic cancer report better symptom severity and physical function than patients with recurrent or metastatic cancer (Siddiqi et al. 2009). Toxicity due to chemotherapy also affects QoL, typically worsening with increasing treatment cycles (Dehkordi et al. 2009). In terminal-stage cancer, the primary treatment goal shifts from curing the disease to optimising QoL (Jocham et al. 2006).

Individual QoL is a subjective perception of physical and mental wellbeing influenced by health risks and conditions, functional status, social support, and socioeconomic status (Centers for Disease Control and Prevention 2021). The European Organisation for the Research and Treatment of Cancer (EORTC) has developed a core 30-item QoL questionnaire (QLQ-C30) for the assessment of health-related QoL of cancer patients. The QLQ-C30 consists of multi-item scales: functional scales for the physical, role, emotional, cognitive, and social functioning; symptom scales for fatigue, pain, nausea, and vomiting; and overall health and QoL scale (Fayers and Bottomley 2002). Another widely used cancer-specific QoL questionnaire is the Functional Assessment of Cancer Therapy-General (FACT-G) (Cella et al. 1993). This 27-item questionnaire evaluates various QoL domains, including physical, functional, family, social, and emotional. Summation of the items provides scores for each domain and an overall QoL score (Webster et al. 2003). A meta-review by Smith et al. (2014) found 55% of oncological randomised controlled trials (RCTs) reporting QoL of cancer patients used either QLQ-C30 or FACT-G as the instrument of measure. These instruments quantify the subjective QoL with patients' reported outcomes for cancer research.

8.2 Disease Mechanisms Affecting QoL

Even though QoL is a subjective construct based on a patient's experience, immunological dysfunction leading to inflammatory processes is an underlying mechanism that causes the cancer patient's reduced physical and emotional status and indirectly impacts social functioning. Hence, there is a call for targeting inflammation in cancer prevention and therapy research.

8.2.1 Systemic Inflammation

Inflammation is a hallmark of cancer, and it is associated with almost all tumour sites (Mantovani et al. 2008; Colotta et al. 2009). Chronic inflammation creates a pro-tumorigenic microenvironment via the production of pro-inflammatory cytokines, angiogenesis, and tissue remodelling. The inflammatory process aids the proliferation and survival of malignant cells, suppressing the adaptive immune response while promoting metastasis (Liu et al. 2015). The release of pro-inflammatory mediators at the surrounding tissues stimulates the recruitment of leukocytes, macrophages, and platelets to enhance the local immune response. Local inflammatory mediators will eventually leak into the circulatory pathways and seed a systemic inflammatory cascade (McAllister and Weinberg 2014).

Systemic inflammation is evident with an increase of circulating white blood cells and an elevation of acute-phase proteins, including C-reactive protein (CRP), haptoglobin, and serum amyloid A. Prolonged systemic inflammation can negatively impact the treatment outcome in both early and advanced cancer (Roxburgh and Mcmillan 2014). Measurements of systemic inflammatory response based on CRP and albumin, together with the modified Glasgow Prognostic Score and various inflammatory-nutritional indexes, show predictive values for cancer survival independent of tumour site and stages (Pastore et al. 2013; Proctor et al. 2011; Peng et al. 2017; Li et al. 2018; Zhang et al. 2017). Hence, systematic inflammation is a vital underlying mechanism leading to poor prognostic outcomes in advanced cancer (McSorley et al. 2017).

An analysis of the QLQ-C30 data collected from a large cohort of 1466 advanced cancer patients across Europe demonstrated a clear relationship between systemic inflammation and QoL (Laird et al. 2013). Increased CRP levels correlated significantly ($p < 0.001$) with global QoL score, performance status, survival, pain, anorexia, cognitive dysfunction, dyspnoea, and fatigue, in addition to physical, social, and role dysfunctions (Laird et al. 2013). A more recent analysis of QLQ-C30 data from 2520 patients with advanced cancer further corroborates a consistent relationship between increasing systemic inflammation and worsening of all QLQ-C30 parameters (Laird et al. 2016). Boen et al. (2018) also reported that cancer patients ($n = 1004$) who had higher social support satisfaction were showing lower levels of inflammation as measured by CRP ($p = 0.09$), interleukin (IL)-6 ($p = 0.11$), and tumour necrosis factor (TNF)-α ($p = 0.025$).

Some smaller studies have also reported correlations between different inflammatory biomarkers and QoL symptoms, albeit with less conclusive results. Kwekkeboom et al. (2018) examined the role of stress and inflammation in the symptom cluster of pain, fatigue, and sleep disturbances in advanced cancer ($n = 188$). The study found no significant relationship between CRP and the symptom clusters that affect QoL. Nonetheless, it reported a significant positive relationship ($\beta = 0.2, p = 0.003$) between the pro-inflammatory cytokine TNF-α and symptom cluster distress, which has been shown to interfere with daily life indirectly (Kwekkeboom et al. 2018). Paulsen et al. (2017) examined the relationship between pro-inflammatory cytokines and pain, appetite, and fatigue in advanced cancer ($n = 49$). The study found IL-6 and CRP to have correlations with appetite ($p < 0.01$). Additionally, IL-1 receptor antagonist was shown to correlate with fatigue ($p < 0.01$), (Paulsen et al. 2017).

8.2.2 Behaviour Comorbidities

Cancer patients and survivors often develop behavioural and emotional problems such as depression, anxiety, fatigue, cognitive impairment, and neuropathic pain that adversely affect the QoL. Depression and anxiety affect about 35% and 10% of cancer patients, respectively (Mitchell et al. 2011). Two-thirds of patients with cancer and depression also have clinically significant anxiety symptoms (Mitchell et al. 2011). Depression and anxiety can affect patients throughout their cancer journey, but most prominently during the acute phase of treatment (Pitman et al. 2018). Closely associated with depression and anxiety, fatigue has been reported by patients at diagnosis (40%), under chemotherapy (80%), and during radiation treatment (90%). In advanced cancer, fatigue is one of the most common and disabling symptoms (Brown and Kroenke 2009).

Cognitive impairment, such as deficits in memory, attention, concentration, and executive function, is reported in 30% of patients before chemotherapy. The prevalence increases to 70% in cancer patients during active treatment. Such impairment persists in about 35% of the patients many years post-treatment (Janelsins et al. 2014; Pendergrass et al. 2018). Up to 40% of patients also experienced neuropathic pain caused by nerve damage attributable to cancer or associated treatment (Bennett et al. 2012). Together, these behavioural comorbidities can severely limit functional independence, reduce adherence to cancer treatment, undermine social life, and generate psychosocial stress.

The inflammatory pathway of behavioural comorbidities that leads to lower QoL is shown in Fig. 8.1. Chemotherapy induces necrosis of both tumour and healthy cells. The dying cells release proteins, nucleic acids, purines, and reactive oxygen species, collectively known as damage-associated molecular patterns (DAMPs) (Santos and Pyter 2018). DAMPs are endogenous danger signals that prime cluster of differentiation (CD) 4+ and CD8+ lymphocytes and trigger a robust adaptive immune response against dead cell-associated antigens (Hernandez et al. 2016). This immune response further increases cytokine release, prolongs inflammation, and

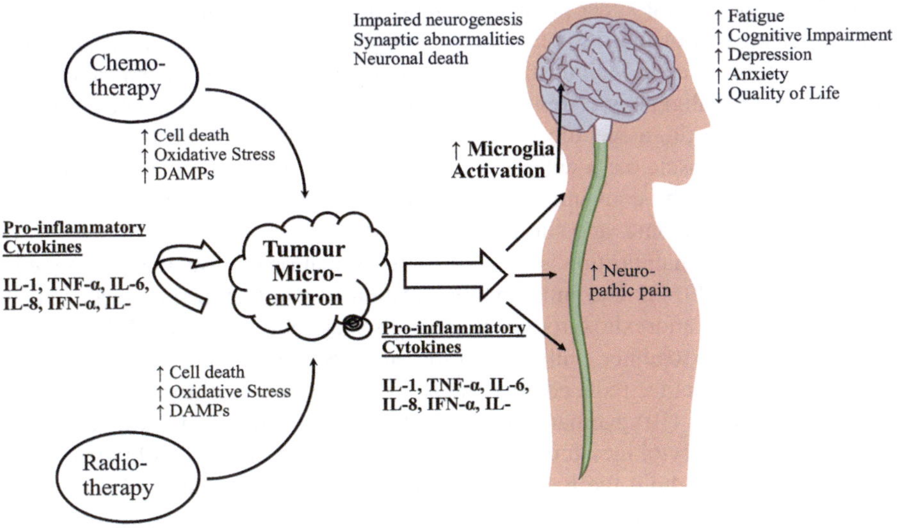

Fig. 8.1 The inflammatory pathway to behavioural comorbidities – adapted from (Santos and Pyter 2018)

contributes to side effects (Santos and Pyter 2018; Hernandez et al. 2016). Chemotherapy toxicity may also weaken the blood-brain barrier, allowing peripheral immune cells to traffic into the brain (Wardill et al. 2016). Similarly, radiotherapy may also induce cell deaths, trigger the release of DAMPs, exacerbate inflammation, and disrupt the immune response (de Carvalho and Villar 2018).

Microglial cells are a specialised population of macrophages in the central nervous system (CNS), and their activation is the cellular source of neuroinflammation. The cumulative inflammatory effects of the tumour microenvironment, chemotherapy, and radiotherapy contribute to microglial activation within the CNS (Santos and Pyter 2018; Sochocka et al. 2017). Neuroinflammation can lead to impaired neurogenesis, synaptic abnormalities, and neuronal death. Damage to the CNS is the cause of behavioural comorbidities and QoL degradation (Santos and Pyter 2018; Sevenich 2018).

8.2.3 Nutritional Status

Malnutrition is a condition associated with significant weight loss and altered body composition due to insufficient intake or uptake of nutrients. It is a cause of diminished physical and mental functions, which also impairs disease outcomes (Cederholm et al. 2017). Cancer-related malnutrition prevalence ranges from 20% to more than 70%, depending on patient age, cancer type, and cancer stage (Arends et al. 2017). In general, older patients are more at risk than younger ones. There is a high prevalence of malnutrition in patients with gastrointestinal tract, head and neck, liver, and lung cancers. Malnutrition is also more common in advanced cancer than in early-stage malignancy (Arends et al. 2017). In severe cases, malnutrition can progress to cachexia, a specific form of malnutrition characterised by the ongoing loss of skeletal muscle mass with or without fat mass loss (Mattox 2017). Cachexia cannot be reversed by conventional nutritional care, and it can dramatically impact QoL, treatment outcome, and survival (Mattox 2017).

Cancer-related malnutrition is also due to the activation of systemic inflammation (Zitvogel et al. 2017). The inflammatory response resulting from cancer and its treatment causes anorexia through altered CNS appetite signals (Molfino et al. 2017). Anorexia, together with symptoms such as nausea, diarrhoea, and pain, leads to poor appetite, reduced food intake, depleted energy stores in fat tissue, and weight loss (Bruggeman et al. 2016). The spread of tumour-derived pro-inflammatory cytokines further disrupts the metabolism of carbohydrates, fats, and proteins throughout the body and reduces nutrient uptake (Schcolnik-Cabrera et al. 2017). Muscle wasting occurs due to ongoing anabolic/catabolic imbalance. This process reduces muscle mass and strength while increasing the level of fatigue (Aversa et al. 2017). Inflammation also stimulates the production of acute-phase proteins in the liver, which represses drug clearance and elevates treatment toxicity risk (Robinson et al. 2016). Pro-inflammatory cytokines can also trigger increased lipid breakdown that causes the defective formation of adipose tissues and lowers the fat mass (Han et al. 2018).

Nutritional status is a significant factor in predicting QoL. Evidence from epidemiological cancer studies shows that patients with better nutritional status generally enjoy better QoL (Lis et al. 2012). For cancer patients requiring only chemotherapy treatment, anorexia, functional impairment, the palliative nature of chemotherapy, and elevated CRP levels are independent predictive factors for reduced QoL (Salas et al. 2017). A cross-sectional study of cancer patients on chemotherapy compared nutritional status to QoL measurement with QLQ-C30 (Vergara et al. 2013). Among the 97 patients, 58 were well-nourished, 32 were moderately malnourished, and 7 were severe malnutrition cases. The study found statistically significant differences ($p < 0.05$) across these groups, according to QLQ-C30 scales of global QoL, physical, role, emotional, and cognitive functioning. The well-nourished group consistently reported better QoL scores in these areas. Furthermore, the well-nourished group also experienced significantly milder ($p < 0.05$) symptoms of fatigue, nausea and vomiting, pain, insomnia, and appetite loss compared to other groups (Vergara et al. 2013).

8.2.4 Targeting Inflammation to Improve QoL

Understanding the role of immuno-inflammatory processes in tumorigenesis has spurred the interest in using natural or biological substances to modify the host immune responses in cancer therapy to reduce side effects, improve outcomes, and enhance QoL (Schirrmacher 2019). These substances are known as biological response modifiers (BRMs) or immunomodulators due to their ability in modulating the antitumour immune response and cancer-related chronic inflammation (Liu et al. 2016; Liao and Oldham 2018; Kuroki et al. 2012). There are two groups of BRMs. The first provides antigen-specific immune responses and may exhibit a direct antitumour effect, such as vaccines and monoclonal antibodies (Kuroki et al. 2012). Anti-inflammatory approaches with monoclonal antibodies that enhance chemotherapy specificity and reduce the severe side effects are now available. However, limitations, including severe adverse effects and high production costs, impede the clinical application (Coulson et al. 2014; Cruz and Kayser 2019).

The second group of immunomodulators consists of the non-specific BRMs, which augment or stimulate the immune system without antigenic specificity (Kuroki et al. 2012). Cytokines are the classical non-specific BRMs. IL-2 and interferon-α are both approved immunotherapies of many cancer types (Lee and Margolin 2011). IL-7, IL-12, IL-15, IL-18, and IL-21 have entered clinical trials with various degrees of success (Liu et al. 2016). However, the use of these BRMs is not without safety issues. Most cytokine therapies carry potentially dangerous side effects concerning neuropsychiatric, autoimmune, ischaemic, and infectious events that may have detrimental effects on the patient's treatment outcome and QoL (Baldo 2014; Davis and Ballas 2017). Hence, research is continuing to seek out novel BRMs that are safe and effective in supporting cancer treatment and improving QoL.

8.3 RBAC for QoL of Cancer Patients

Arabinoxylan is a non-starch polysaccharide found in many cereal grains. It is considered a dietary fibre that can positively impact gut microbial growth and the immune system (Mendis et al. 2016). Rice bran arabinoxylan compound (RBAC) is a specific blend of hemicelluloses extracted from rice bran with enzymes from shiitake mushrooms (*Lentinus edodes* mycelia). Research has shown that RBAC possesses strong immunomodulating properties with clinical applications in cancer treatment (Ooi et al. 2018; Ghoneum 2016). As such, RBAC is used among cancer patients as an immunomodulator to support weakened immune function during and after conventional cancer treatment (Paterson 2002). RBAC has been shown to be a safe and effective plant-based BRM with immunomodulating and anti-inflammatory properties that can improve cancer patients' QoL (Ooi et al. 2018).

8.3.1 Direct and Indirect Pathways

As a non-specific BRM, RBAC modulates the immune and inflammatory responses via both direct and indirect pathways. A portion of the ingested RBAC enters the bloodstream via gut mucosa. It exerts direct effects on innate and adaptive immune activities, including enhanced NK cell immunosurveillance, macrophage

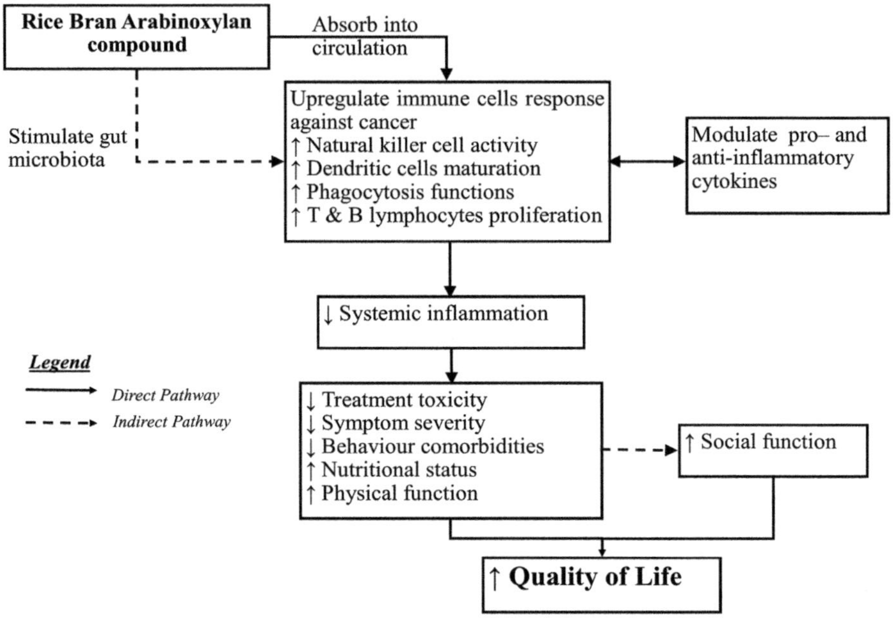

Fig. 8.2 Model showing RBAC influencing the cancer patient QoL via direct (absorption) and indirect (gut microbiota) pathways

phagocytosis, dendritic cell maturation, and B and T lymphocyte proliferation (Ghoneum 2016), with details presented in earlier chapters. The remaining portion of ingested RBAC that is resistant to digestion serves as a prebiotic to gut microbiota. The metabolites released by gut bacteria, such as the short-chain fatty acids (Gu et al. 2020), induce anti-inflammatory and immunomodulating effects in the host (Mendis et al. 2016) and affect behavioural changes via the gut-brain axis (Martin and Mayer 2017).

The improved immune cell activity against cancer by RBAC is shown through both direct and indirect pathways by modulating the balance of pro-inflammatory and anti-inflammatory cytokines and reducing systemic inflammation. Such improvement can have beneficial effects on lowering cancer treatment toxicity, symptom severity, and behavioural comorbidities. Patients may experience improved physical functioning, nutritional status, and, indirectly, enhanced social functioning. The overall cancer patient QoL is thus enhanced. Figure 8.2 is an illustration of how RBAC can influence cancer patient QoL.

8.3.2 Current Evidence

Improved QoL using RBAC among cancer patients has been documented in many case studies (Ooi et al. 2018). The reported benefits include subjective improvement in sleep, appetite, digestion, physical activity, decreased anxiety, pain, and reduced adverse effects during cancer therapy. Notwithstanding, clinical research on RBAC and cancer QoL is at its early stage, with only a small number of clinical trials available in the literature.

The effect of RBAC on QoL of breast cancer patients undergoing adjuvant chemotherapy was studied by Masood et al. (2013) in an RCT with 50 participants. This study found RBAC to improve QoL by reducing tiredness, anti-emetic needs, alopecia, and increased appetite during chemotherapy.

Takahara and Sano (2004) observed the effect of RBAC supplementation on the QoL of locally advanced and metastatic cancer patients after surgery ($n = 205$) in a 6-month RCT. RBAC plus a standardised set of complementary alternative therapies (sCAT) improved appetite better than the sCAT alone (+24.6% vs +15.6%). After 18 months of treatment, 54.2% of the RBAC group survived compared to only 17.4% in the sCAT group. However, no significant tests were reported on these observations.

In Hajtó et al. (2016), 35 cancer patients with various malignancies were treated with a combination of mistletoe lectin and RBAC as immunomodulators during conventional oncotherapy over 6 months. The patients reported their QoL on a customised questionnaire. This single-arm trial reported improved physical activity and decreased side effects ($n = 25$, 71%) as the most important findings of this combined treatment during conventional oncotherapy.

Petrovics et al. (2016) studied the effects of RBAC (3 g/day for 24 weeks) plus oncothermia therapy on cancer patients with different malignancies who suffered from chronic fatigue syndrome (CFS) in an RCT ($n = 50$). RBAC plus oncothermia group showed improvement in CFS symptoms with a significant reduction in the mean fatigue scale ($p < 0.05$).

Tan and Flores (2020) reported the effects of RBAC on the QoL for head and neck carcinoma patients in a recent RCT. Sixty-five patients were randomly assigned to receive either RBAC or placebo (3 g/day) as an adjuvant for radiation therapy in a double-blind RCT. Patients receiving RBAC reported significantly higher haematologic parameters, lower treatment-related toxicity grading, and higher QoL scores measured with the EORTC H & N35 questionnaire than control ($p = 0.019$). These outcomes resulted in less blood transfusion, treatment delays, and hospital admissions among RBAC patients. The study also noted that 11 patients died during treatment, with none from the RBAC group. Hence, supplementation with RBAC resulted in higher QoL and better clinical outcomes.

8.4 Future Directions

Increasing importance in cancer treatment is now placed on achieving benefits in cancer patients' QoL, in addition to survival. RBAC can improve the QoL of cancer patients through its immunomodulating and anti-inflammatory properties. The mounting evidence on the effect of RBAC for QoL of cancer patients supports its use as a complementary therapy in cancer management.

However, existing research suffers from several limitations, including inadequate study design with unclear risks of bias as well as the use of non-validated QoL measurements (Ooi et al. 2020). Furthermore, placebo treatment is well known to positively affect the QoL of cancer patients, especially in improved control of symptoms such as pain, appetite, and fatigue but rarely with positive tumour response (Hoenemeyer et al. 2018; Chvetzoff and Tannock 2003). Most published trials did not attempt to rule out the impact of placebo effects in the QoL improvement observed with RBAC supplementation. Hence, comparing the clinical effects of RBAC on the cancer patient QoL with placebo as the control comparator is essential to ascertain the real effects of RBAC.

Additionally, most existing RBAC studies did not measure cancer patients' systemic inflammation, cytokine response, and nutritional status while assessing their QoL. Also, how RBAC may affect QoL via the gut microbiota needs further investigation. A new placebo-controlled RCT is currently underway to address these limitations and assess the effects of RBAC on cancer patients' QoL with the validated QLQ-C30 questionnaires (Ooi et al. 2020).

Research has shown that circulating tumour cells (CTC) can be a useful prognostic marker for cancer metastasis (Lin et al. 2021). In a recently reported case series, RBAC has been shown to significantly lower ($p = 0.0047$, $n = 14$) the CTC levels of a group of patients with prostate, breast, uterine, or ovarian cancer (Pescatore et al. 2022). With metastatic cancer being the critical factor influencing QoL, future research investigating RBAC and cancer QoL may consider CTC as the objective biomarker to correlate with the changes in subjective patient-reported outcome measures. This topic will continue to be an active area of research.

References

Arends J, Baracos V, Bertz H, Bozzetti F, Calder PC, Deutz NEP et al (2017) ESPEN expert group recommendations for action against cancer-related malnutrition. Clin Nutr 36:1187–1196

Aversa Z, Costelli P, Muscaritoli M (2017) Cancer-induced muscle wasting: latest findings in prevention and treatment. Ther Adv Med Oncol 9:369–382

Baldo BA (2014) Side effects of cytokines approved for therapy. Drug Saf 37:921–943

Bennett M, Rayment C, Hjermstad M, Aass N, Caraceni A, Kaasa S (2012) Prevalence and aetiology of neuropathic pain in cancer patients: a systematic review. Pain 153:359–365

Boen CE, Barrow DA, Bensen JT, Farnan L, Gerstel A, Hendrix LH et al (2018) Social relationships, inflammation, and cancer survival. Cancer Epidemiol Biomark Prev 27:541–549

Brown LF, Kroenke K (2009) Cancer-related fatigue and its associations with depression and anxiety: a systematic review. Psychosomatics 50:440–447

Bruggeman AR, Kamal AH, LeBlanc TW, Ma JD, Baracos VE, Roeland EJ (2016) Cancer cachexia: beyond weight loss. J Oncol Pract 12:1163–1171

Cederholm T, Barazzoni R, Austin P, Ballmer P, Biolo G, Bischoff SC et al (2017) ESPEN guidelines on definitions and terminology of clinical nutrition. Clin Nutr 36:49–64

Cella D, Tulsky D, Gray G, Sarafian B, Linn E, Bonomi A et al (1993) The functional assessment of cancer therapy scale: development and validation of the general measure. J Clin Oncol 11:570–579

Centers for Disease Control and Prevention (2021) HRQOL concepts [Internet]. [cited 2021 Feb 22]. https://www.cdc.gov/hrqol/concept.htm

Chvetzoff G, Tannock I (2003) Placebo effects in oncology. J Natl Cancer Inst 95:19–29
Colotta F, Allavena P, Sica A, Garlanda C, Mantovani A (2009) Cancer-related inflammation, the seventh hallmark of cancer: links to genetic instability. Carcinogenesis 30:1073–1081
Coulson A, Levy A, Gossell-Williams M (2014) Monoclonal antibodies in cancer therapy: mechanisms, successes and limitations. West Indian Med J 63:650–654
Cruz E, Kayser V (2019) Monoclonal antibody therapy of solid tumors: clinical limitations and novel strategies to enhance treatment efficacy. Biologics 13:33–51
Davis BP, Ballas ZK (2017) Biologic response modifiers: indications, implications, and insights. J Allergy Clin Immunol 139:1445–1456
de Carvalho HA, Villar RC (2018) Radiotherapy and immune response: the systemic effects of a local treatment. Clinics (Sao Paulo) 73:e557s
Dehkordi A, Heydarnejad MS, Fatehi D (2009) Quality of life in cancer patients undergoing chemotherapy. Oman Med J 24:204–207
Fayers P, Bottomley A (2002) Quality of life research within the EORTC—the EORTC QLQ-C30. Eur J Cancer 38:125–133
Ghoneum M (2016) From bench to bedside: the growing use of arabinoxylan rice bran (MGN-3/Biobran) in cancer immunotherapy. Austin Immunol 1:1006
Gu I, Lam WS, Marasini D, Brownmiller C, Savary B, Lee JA et al (2020) In vitro fecal fermentation patterns of arabinoxylan from rice bran on gut microbiota in normal weight and overweight/obese subjects. Curr Dev Nutr 4:1560
Hajtó T, Horvath A, Papp S (2016) Improvement of quality of life in tumor patients after an immunomodulatory treatment with standardized mistletoe lectin and arabinoxylan plant extracts. Int J Neurorehabil 3:2–4
Han J, Meng Q, Shen L, Wu G (2018) Interleukin-6 induces fat loss in cancer cachexia by promoting white adipose tissue lipolysis and browning. Lipids Health Dis 17:14
Hernandez C, Huebener P, Schwabe RF (2016) Damage-associated molecular patterns in cancer: a double-edged sword. Oncogene 35:5931–5941
Hoenemeyer TW, Kaptchuk TJ, Mehta TS, Fontaine KR (2018) Open-label placebo treatment for cancer-related fatigue: a randomized-controlled clinical trial. Sci Rep 8:2784
Janelsins MC, Kesler SR, Ahles TA, Morrow GR (2014) Prevalence, mechanisms, and management of cancer-related cognitive impairment. Int Rev Psychiatry 26:102–113
Jocham HR, Dassen T, Widdershoven G, Halfens R (2006) Quality of life in palliative care cancer patients: a literature review. J Clin Nurs 15:1188–1195
Kuroki M, Miyamoto S, Morisaki T, Yotsumoto F, Shirasu N, Taniguchi Y et al (2012) Biological response modifiers used in cancer biotherapy. Anticancer Res 32:2229–2233
Kwekkeboom KL, Tostrud L, Costanzo E, Coe CL, Serlin RC, Ward SE et al (2018) The role of inflammation in the pain, fatigue, and sleep disturbance symptom cluster in advanced cancer. J Pain Symptom Manag 55:1286–1295
Laird BJA, McMillan DC, Fayers P, Fearon K, Kaasa S, Fallon MT et al (2013) The systemic inflammatory response and its relationship to pain and other symptoms in advanced cancer. Oncologist 18:1050–1055
Laird BJA, Fallon M, Hjermstad MJ, Tuck S, Kaasa S, Klepstad P et al (2016) Quality of life in patients with advanced cancer: differential association with performance status and systemic inflammatory response. J Clin Oncol 34:2769–2775
Lee S, Margolin K (2011) Cytokines in cancer immunotherapy. Cancers (Basel) 3:3856–3893
Li D, Yuan X, Liu J, Li C, Li W (2018) Prognostic value of prognostic nutritional index in lung cancer: a meta-analysis. J Thorac Dis 10:5298–5307
Liao S-K, Oldham RK (2018) Immunotherapy of cancer is a part of biotherapy. J Cancer Metastasis Treat 4:3
Lin D, Shen L, Luo M et al (2021) Circulating tumor cells: biology and clinical significance. Signal Transduct Target Ther 6:404
Lis CG, Gupta D, Lammersfeld CA, Markman M, Vashi PG (2012) Role of nutritional status in predicting quality of life outcomes in cancer--a systematic review of the epidemiological literature. Nutr J 11:27

Liu J, Lin PC, Zhou BP (2015) Inflammation fuels tumor progress and metastasis. Curr Pharm Des 21:3032–3040

Liu R, Luo F, Liu X, Wang L, Yang J, Deng Y et al (2016) Biological response modifier in cancer immunotherapy. Adv Exp Med Biol 909:69–138

Mantovani A, Allavena P, Sica A, Balkwill F (2008) Cancer-related inflammation. Nature 454:436–444

Martin CR, Mayer EA (2017) Gut-brain axis and behavior. Nestle Nutr Inst Workshop Ser 88:45–53

Masood AI, Sheikh R, Anwer RA (2013) "BIOBRAN MGN-3"; effect of reducing side effects of chemotherapy in breast cancer patients. Prof Med J 20:13–16

Mattox TW (2017) Cancer cachexia: cause, diagnosis, and treatment. Nutr Clin Pract 32:599–606

McAllister SS, Weinberg RA (2014) The tumour-induced systemic environment as a critical regulator of cancer progression and metastasis. Nat Cell Biol 16:717–727

McSorley ST, Dolan RD, Roxburgh CSD, McMillan DC, Horgan PG (2017) How and why systemic inflammation worsens quality of life in patients with advanced cancer. Expert Rev Qual Life Cancer Care 2:167–175

Mendis M, Leclerc E, Simsek S (2016) Arabinoxylans, gut microbiota and immunity. Carbohydr Polym 139:159–166

Mitchell AJ, Chan M, Bhatti H, Halton M, Grassi L, Johansen C et al (2011) Prevalence of depression, anxiety, and adjustment disorder in oncological, haematological, and palliative-care settings: a meta-analysis of 94 interview-based studies. Lancet Oncol 12:160–174

Molfino A, Iannace A, Colaiacomo MC, Farcomeni A, Emiliani A, Gualdi G et al (2017) Cancer anorexia: hypothalamic activity and its association with inflammation and appetite-regulating peptides in lung cancer. J Cachexia Sarcopenia Muscle 8:40–47

Ooi SL, McMullen D, Golombick T, Pak SC (2018) Evidence-based review of BioBran/MGN-3 arabinoxylan compound as a complementary therapy for conventional cancer treatment. Integr Cancer Ther 17:165–178

Ooi SL, Pak SC, Micalos PS, Schupfer E, Zielinski R, Jeffries T et al (2020) Rice bran arabinoxylan compound and quality of life of cancer patients (RBAC-QoL): study protocol for a randomized pilot feasibility trial. Contemp Clin Trials Commun 19:100580

Pastore CA, González MC, Orlandi SP (2013) Association between an inflammatory-nutritional index and nutritional status in cancer patients. Nutr Hosp 28:188–193

Paterson A (2002) Therapeutic properties of biobran MGN-3. Posit Heal [Internet]. http://www.positivehealth.com/article/nutraceuticals/therapeutic-properties-of-biobran-mgn-3

Paulsen Ø, Laird B, Aass N, Lea T, Fayers P, Kaasa S et al (2017) The relationship between pro-inflammatory cytokines and pain, appetite and fatigue in patients with advanced cancer. PLoS One 12:e0177620

Pendergrass JC, Targum SD, Harrison JE (2018) Cognitive impairment associated with cancer: a brief review. Innov Clin Neurosci 15:36–44

Peng J, Zhang R, Zhao Y, Wu X, Chen G, Wan D et al (2017) Prognostic value of preoperative prognostic nutritional index and its associations with systemic inflammatory response markers in patients with stage III colon cancer. Chin J Cancer 36:96

Pescatore F, Prestano C, Kichikova M (2022) RBAC and its role with the immune system. Altern Ther Health Med 28:8–10

Petrovics G, Szigeti G, Hamvas S, Máté Á, Betlehem J, Hegyi G (2016) Controlled pilot study for cancer patients suffering from chronic fatigue syndrome due to chemotherapy treated with BioBran (MGN-3-Arabinoxylane) and targeted radiofrequency heat therapy. Eur J Integr Med 8:29–35

Pitman A, Suleman S, Hyde N, Hodgkiss A (2018) Depression and anxiety in patients with cancer. BMJ 361:k1415

Proctor MJ, Morrison DS, Talwar D, Balmer SM, Fletcher CD, O'Reilly DSJ et al (2011) A comparison of inflammation-based prognostic scores in patients with cancer. A Glasgow inflammation outcome study. Eur J Cancer 47:2633–2641

Robinson MW, Harmon C, O'Farrelly C (2016) Liver immunology and its role in inflammation and homeostasis. Cell Mol Immunol 13:267–276

Roxburgh CSD, Mcmillan DC (2014) Cancer and systemic inflammation: treat the tumour and treat the host. Br J Cancer 110:1409–1412

Salas S, Mercier S, Moheng B, Olivet S, Garcia M-E, Hamon S et al (2017) Nutritional status and quality of life of cancer patients needing exclusive chemotherapy: a longitudinal study. Health Qual Life Outcomes 15:85

Santos JC, Pyter LM (2018) Neuroimmunology of behavioral comorbidities associated with cancer and cancer treatments. Front Immunol 9:1195

Schcolnik-Cabrera A, Chávez-Blanco A, Domínguez-Gómez G, Dueñas-González A (2017) Understanding tumor anabolism and patient catabolism in cancer-associated cachexia. Am J Cancer Res 7:1107–1135

Schirrmacher V (2019) From chemotherapy to biological therapy: a review of novel concepts to reduce the side effects of systemic cancer treatment (review). Int J Oncol 54:407–419

Sevenich L (2018) Brain-resident microglia and blood-borne macrophages orchestrate central nervous system inflammation in neurodegenerative disorders and brain cancer. Front Immunol 9:697

Siddiqi A, Given CW, Given B, Sikorskii A (2009) Quality of life among patients with primary, metastatic and recurrent cancer. Eur J Cancer Care (Engl) 18:84–96

Smith A, Cocks K, Parry D, Taylor M (2014) Reporting of health-related quality of life (HRQOL) data in oncology trials: a comparison of the European Organization for Research and Treatment of Cancer Quality of Life (EORTC QLQ-C30) and the Functional Assessment of Cancer Therapy-General (FACT-G). Qual Life Res 23:971–976

Sochocka M, Diniz BS, Leszek J (2017) Inflammatory response in the CNS: friend or foe? Mol Neurobiol 54:8071–8089

Takahara K, Sano K (2004) Life prolongation and QOL improvement effect of modified arabinoxylan from rice bran (BioBran/MGN-3) for progressive cancer. Clin Pharmacol Ther 14:267–271

Tan DFS, Flores JAS (2020) The immunomodulating effects of arabinoxylan rice bran (Lentin) on hematologic profile, nutritional status and quality of life among head and neck carcinoma patients undergoing radiation therapy: a double blind randomized control trial. Radiol J Off Publ Philip Coll Radiol 12(February):11–16

Vergara N, Montoya JE, Luna HG, Amparo JR, Cristal-Luna G (2013) Quality of life and nutritional status among cancer patients on chemotherapy. Oman Med J 28:270–274

Wardill HR, Mander KA, Van Sebille YZA, Gibson RJ, Logan RM, Bowen JM et al (2016) Cytokine-mediated blood brain barrier disruption as a conduit for cancer/chemotherapy-associated neurotoxicity and cognitive dysfunction. Int J Cancer 139:2635–2645

Webster K, Cella D, Yost K (2003) The functional assessment of chronic illness therapy (FACIT) measurement system: properties, applications, and interpretation. Health Qual Life Outcomes 1: 79

World Health Organization (2021) WHOQOL: measuring quality of life [Internet]. [cited 2021 Feb 22]. https://www.who.int/tools/whoqol

Zhang W, Ye B, Liang W, Ren Y (2017) Preoperative prognostic nutritional index is a powerful predictor of prognosis in patients with stage III ovarian cancer. Sci Rep 7:9548

Zitvogel L, Pietrocola F, Kroemer G (2017) Nutrition, inflammation and cancer. Nat Immunol 18: 843

Part IV

Applications in Other Conditions

Part IV aims at exploring the potential use of RBAC in different medical conditions, and each includes the scientific evidence behind it.

Chronic Microinflammation as "Friendly-Fire" in Aging and Disease

9

Yuzo Endo, Kentaro Ninomiya, and Soo Liang Ooi

Abstract

Major lifestyle-related chronic diseases, including cancer and Alzheimer's disease, are the consequences of long-term micro-inflammation in any microenvironment in our body with a latency of 10–20 years. Inflammation is an immune response triggered by leucocytes, such as macrophages and neutrophils, producing and spreading reactive oxygen species in response not only to pathogens but also to self-structural substances, even DNA. Such oxidative stress affects host cells, so-called friendly-fire. One of the worthiest preventive strategies for lifestyle-related diseases is suppression or downregulation of friendly-fire attacks not by drugs but by potent food supplements. Research conducted by the lead author has confirmed the partially absorbed Biobran with its derivatives in mouse blood after oral intake. The uptake of Biobran may be through Peyer's patches in the small intestines. Further experimentation also demonstrated that both oral intake and parenteral administration of Biobran in mice induced comparable protective effects against the adverse effects of anticancer drugs, which are potent oxidants and even carcinogenic. Hence, the antioxidant, immunomodulating, and anti-inflammatory effects of BioBran can attenuate the "friendly-fire" in lifestyle-related chronic diseases in adulthood and aging.

Y. Endo (✉)
Hamamatsu University School of Medicine, Hamamatsu, Japan

K. Ninomiya
Daiwa Pharmaceutical Co., Ltd., Tokyo, Japan

S. L. Ooi
School of Dentistry and Medical Sciences, Charles Sturt University, Bathurst, NSW, Australia

S. C. Pak et al. (eds.), *Modified Rice Bran Arabinoxylan*,
https://doi.org/10.1007/978-981-19-5735-2_9

Keywords

Evidence-based · Oral supplement · Biobran · Antioxidant · Immune modulation · Lifestyle diseases · Preventive medicine

9.1 Introduction

Many diseases in humans are now recognized as chronic inflammatory processes initiated and promoted by lifestyle factors. Chronic inflammatory diseases can take as long as 15–20 years of latency before symptoms appear. After which, they can progress rapidly and reach the end stage without proper treatment. Major lifestyle-related chronic diseases include cancer, diabetes mellitus, obesity-related diseases, and atherosclerosis which can lead to ischemic diseases in the heart and the brain and Alzheimer's disease. This lifestyle etiology aspect is revolutionarily different from the traditional pathological viewpoint until the late twentieth century.

Aging is physiological life with eustress, whereas senescence is pathological life with distress. A balance of eustress and distress regulates a healthy life. In a review paper on aging published in 2000, Franceschi et al. presented the inflamm-aging theory, an epoch-making and groundbreaking concept in modern medical sciences (Franceschi et al. 2000). Aging and chronic microinflammation must be considered based on minute repeating oxidative stress produced by the host's inflammatory cells, such as leucocytes, against foreign pathogens and own cells (Endo et al. 1993). The process is akin to "friendly-fire" as a simile. The causes of chronic diseases consist of glycation by glucose over-intake, lipid over-intake, and nitrogen imbalance leading to amyloid deposition, even though these are fundamental nutrients required for cellular energy production. Deoxyribonucleic acid (DNA)-ribonucleic acid (RNA)-protein biosynthesis, the central dogma of molecular biology, is one of the most important targets of lifestyle-related disease.

BioBran is a type of modified arabinoxylan hemicellulose compound derived from rice bran. It has been established as a nontoxic supplement called a biological response modifier (BRM) that can trigger immunogenic responses (Ghoneum 2016). With its antioxidant and immunomodulatory effects, BioBran can protect against lifestyle-related disease holistically.

As a diagnostic pathologist and clinical immunologist in the Toranomon General Hospital in Tokyo, I (the first author) conducted over 700 autopsy cases. I have diagnosed clinical biopsies of the liver, kidney, and other surgical materials for clinicians and patients. I officially reported the final diagnosis with complete comments and published many scientific papers.

I started researching into BioBran using animal models just after I retired from the hospital. I wanted to know the intracorporeal dynamics of BioBran. Since plant compounds are foreign substances to the immune system, I wanted to know how BioBran as a plant-derived arabinoxylan compound affected the animal body after oral intake or parenteral administration. I wanted to know the immunological mechanisms of its cellular and intracellular interaction in terms of novel plant substances in the animal body. Arabinoxylan hemicellulose is a unique and immune-reactive substance in the body from an immunological perspective.

Regarding these questions, contributions by Ghoneum (2016) clarified multiple functions of BioBran, including activation of natural killer (NK) cells and its anti-inflammatory, antioxidant, anticancer, and immunomodulatory effects. These results reveal that BioBran is an ideal BRM derived from foodstuff, in this case, rice bran.

Above all, a couple of papers greatly impressed me. First, a clinical case study showed prolonged survival of the patient with malignant hemangiopericytoma who only took BioBran after surgery (Markus et al. 2006). Second, a recent review article by Ooi et al. documented the evidence-based complementary or alternative therapy using BioBran for conventional cancer treatment (Ooi et al. 2018). These papers show the multifaceted functions of BioBran, affirming its recommendation as adjuvant anticancer therapy and an immune checkpoint therapy. Moreover, BioBran should be recommended to people with lifestyle diseases and those interested in preventing the senescence of aging due to its immunomodulatory effects.

9.2 Trace Experiments of BioBran In Vivo

The best dietary supplement is a substance that will reach the microenvironment in our body and vividly perform crosstalk with cells, tissues, and organ systems, such as the immune, autonomic nervous, and endocrine. These three systems are the basic balancing system of the body's natural healing power. BioBran is an ideal substance for this purpose.

Regarding my first question about BioBran, it must be absorbed into the body to react with the immune system. Thus, trace experiments of BioBran in animals should be done. For tracing BioBran, we developed immunological semiquantitative methods by using polyclonal antibodies against arabinoxylan hemicellulose. We injected crude BioBran into rats that developed polyclonal antibodies against BioBran, which comprises polysaccharides and proteins. In general, polysaccharides show relatively weak antigenicity compared to proteins (Endo and Kanbayashi 2003).

In 2000, while I was a visiting professor at McMaster University, we utilized a then newly developed non-isotopic micro-detection method based on enzyme-linked immunosorbent assay (ELISA) to detect polysaccharide antigens (Zielen et al. 1996). First, we purified polyclonal immunoglobulin (Ig) G antibodies against BioBran compound in experimental rats. We wanted to know if these antibodies could react with mice's sera through oral or intraperitoneal administration of BioBran. In this procedure, BioBran was given to mice orally for digestion through the gut. We expected no trace elements in mice's blood would be detected; however, that was not the case.

Each serum of the experimental groups was incubated with the standard titer of polyclonal IgG antibodies against BioBran. These samples were then ultracentrifuged, and the supernatant with remaining BioBran was tested to react with the serum of standard IgG antibodies against BioBran. Sera without BioBran should show 100% of polyclonal IgG antibodies against BioBran. If some BioBran in sera was present, then antigen-antibody complexes should be precipitated by ultracentrifugation, and some percentage less than 100% of polyclonal IgG antibodies against BioBran would be detected. That means the subtraction of precipitation of antigen of BioBran compound and these antibodies against BioBran (Endo and Kanbayashi 2003).

We detected compound molecules of immunoreactive polysaccharides and proteins of BioBran on the CovaLink ELISA plates, which showed that BioBran could not be fully digested in the gut. A portion was absorbed through the gut, such as through Peyer's patches in the experimental mice, with oral intake of BioBran. We detected immunoreactive BioBran in sera 2 and 3 h later. These results led us to conclude that BioBran can only be partially digested in the gut and absorbed into the blood (Endo and Kanbayashi 2003). Such data of oral intake of drugs or supplements should be necessary to evaluate the dynamics of them in vivo and in humans.

After this, we set up additional mice experiments of oral and intraperitoneal administration of BioBran. We evaluated the protective effect of BioBran against the adverse complication of cisplatin, an anticancer drug. All groups of mice revealed almost the same weight gain pattern for a week after intraperitoneal cisplatin administration. However, the two groups on BioBran (oral and intraperitoneal) showed less weight loss and recovered faster than the control groups on water against cisplatin-induced body weight loss (Endo and Kanbayashi 2003).

Then, we used other animal models to show the protective effects of BioBran against adverse reactions of other anticancer drugs. We developed animal models of acute interstitial pneumonia with anticancer drugs and bronchial asthma (Kanbayashi and Endo 2002). Our work was followed by the in vitro experiment of bone-derived mast cells with hydrolyzed rice bran fraction of BioBran done by Hoshino et al. (2010). The results indicated that BioBran had the potential anti-allergic effect in suppressing degranulation and histamine release from basophils and mast cells.

The large molecular size of BioBran is known to have anticancer effects by upregulating the activities of NK cells, T cells, B cells, and macrophages and by inducing apoptosis of cancer cells (Ghoneum and Abedi 2004). These animal experiments showed that BioBran could protect significantly against inflammatory infiltration and allergic reactions in terms of downregulation of histamine release from mast cells in vivo (Hoshino et al. 2010). Mechanisms of the subcellular action of BioBran should be further analyzed and recognized to understand its immunomodulatory and antioxidant effects.

9.3 Oxidants Attack as Friendly-Fire Causing Inflammation in Lifestyle-Related Disease and Aging

Through autopsies in the hospital, I recognized that almost all adult cancer cases progressed through a long latency period of more than 15 years to appear as solid tumors of more than 1 cm^3 detectable as early-stage cancers. Cancers in adulthood are significantly different from those in children. In adults, this includes cancers of the lung, colon, stomach, esophagus, pancreas, urinary bladder, and breast in females or prostate in males. In children, this includes leukemia, brain tumor, or some blastomas, such as Wilms' tumor. In general, the two groups are quite different from each other.

We already know how the differences between cancer in adulthood and childhood occur. Carcinogenesis in adulthood is closely related to lifestyle. Carcinogenesis in children is closely related to the DNA mutation during the growth of organs in utero. Multiple steps of carcinogenesis are due to spontaneous mutations or methylations of base pairs in the areas of exons related to genes of cellular proliferation, cellular inhibition, apoptosis, or telomeres. Although causes of large-scale mutations remain to be clarified, the etiology of cancer in adulthood is closely related to lifestyle, such as cigarette smoking or inhalation of polluted gasses containing polyaromatic hydrocarbon asbestos, in terms of cancer in the respiratory tract and the pleura. These substances must enter through the lung into the blood, causing changes in the oxidative reactions in our body. They are then excreted through all glands, such as the stomach, breast, pancreas, prostate, urinary tract, and bladder. On the other hand, plant substances, such as vegetables and fruits, grow in fields under the sun's electromagnetic beams, which induce strong oxidative reactions. Plants cannot grow without leaves, which have abundant antioxidants against the sun's radiation.

While I was a visiting professor of mucosal immunology at McMaster University, I was interviewed by Simon Martin, the Complementary and Alternative Medicine (CAM) magazine editor. The article was entitled "Cancer and inflammation: the potential for prevention" and appeared in Vol 4 of August 2004 (Endo 2004). At that time, this information in the interview was speculative. However, since then, the information appears to be correct. I mentioned the following about BioBran.

According to Ariel's paper, cancer growth of the lungs and bronchi was not present until 1912 (Ariel et al. 1950). Later, coal tar or coal smoke was used in animal experiments. In 1917, Professor Yamagiwa published a paper on carcinogenesis by coal tar on rabbits' ears, which was the first chemical carcinogenesis experiment in the world (Fujiki 2014). Coal and cigarette tar are almost the same carcinogenic, phlogistic (inflammation causing) substances with high amounts of oxidants (Seelig and Benignus 1936).

9.4 Tobacco and Cigarettes as a Model of the Initiator and Promoter of Carcinogenesis

Cigarette smoking is a causative factor of carcinogenesis, not tobacco alone. The traditional use of tobacco is quite different from modern-day smoking of cigarettes. Native Americans have sniffed, smoked, chewed, ate, drank (like tea), and smeared tobacco over bodies for medicinal and religious purpose for millennials before the arrival of Christopher Columbus (Musk and de Klerk 2003). Tobacco is still used in tribal ceremonies in South America today. Tobacco smoking was customized by the

Europeans in the fifteenth century throughout the world. The machine producing cigarette was invented in the nineteenth century in France and then spread throughout the world. The mass production and marketing of cigarettes has encouraged tobacco abuse and nicotine addiction (Musk and de Klerk 2003).

When cigarette smoke is inhaled, irritable substances such as tar repeatedly attack moving microvilli of the bronchial epithelium until reaching the alveolar space, leading to cell damage. Then arachidonic acids from the cellular membrane composed of glycerophospholipid release to cause the eicosanoid cascade to occur, resulting in microinflammation around the erosive foci of the mucous membrane of the respiratory tracts (Lee et al. 2012). Within this area, called the microenvironment, macrophages and neutrophils infiltrate to produce and release a substantial oxidative load. These oxidants attack not only foreign substances such as bacteria but also host cells, as friendly-fire that attack the repairing epithelial DNA. Damage of DNA exons can reach the point of no return in the mutations within epithelial DNA. The process starts from the premalignant stage of squamous metaplasia and then becomes malignant (Hecht 2012). Almost all processes of cancer formation in adulthood are like this. However, BioBran can prevent friendly-fire and avoid microinflammation. BioBran should be taken for the antioxidant and anti-inflammatory effects to prevent and protect against fundamental processes of carcinogenesis, not only in the lung but also in other organs mentioned below.

Chemoprevention through dietary supplements, acupuncture, homeopathy, aroma, or other complementary techniques has broad support in the scientific literature. That means that cancer in adulthood could be prevented and treated. Primary prevention is dependent upon protection against oxidant attacks. Secondary prevention is supported by modern medicine through early detection and early treatment. Tertiary prevention for patients in advanced cancer stages must be supported by medical treatments as much as possible, including target-oriented, evidence-based dietary supplements.

9.5 Cancer in the Upper Digestive Tract

The friendly-fire processes mentioned above occur in the oral cavity through chewing betel nuts in Southeast Asia (Sharan et al. 2012) and in the esophagus by drinking hot water such as coffee and sake, leading to a heat-denatured epithelium and then a repairing of the epithelium attacked by the host's inflammatory cells (Loomis et al. 2016). The esophageal epithelium can be eroded by high-percentage alcohols (Liu et al. 2015), such as whiskey or dry gin, and cigarette smoking (Hecht 2012). BioBran should be taken to counteract these cases for its anti-inflammatory and antioxidant effects.

Sodium chloride (NaCl) is the major cause of gastric carcinogenesis through atrophic gastritis or intestinal metaplasia as precancer atypia of the fundic gland zone (Wang et al. 2009). NaCl attacks powerfully to damage the mucosal barrier, which normally protects the stomach epithelium against lowered pH by hydrochloric acid (HCl). HCl in the gastric juice is also a strong acid that attacks the gastric epithelium.

A stress ulcer of the stomach by vagus nerve stimulation is also a promoting factor in becoming an erosion or ulcer. Repeated erosions of the gastric mucosa by NaCl and HCl cause atrophic changes of the fundic glands leading to an atrophic condition in a nonacidic environment. The stomach's intraluminal environment shows a higher pH, such as around neutral, where *Helicobacter pylori* can grow and infect erosive mucosa with inflammation. *H. pylori* appears to be one of the most important bystanders of the microinflammatory processes of gastric cancer (Gaddy et al. 2013).

The antral area in the stomach is a common site of gastric cancer because it is easy to become erosive during a microinflammatory response. The infiltration of macrophages and leukocytes produces reactive oxygen radicals against infection and to repair epithelial cells. This initiates a friendly-fire attack to repair the DNA of gastric epithelial cells.

The incidence of gastric cancer in the United States was high before the Second World War. At that time, NaCl and nitric acids were mainly used as additives for food storage. After electric refrigerators were invented and sold, consumption of NaCl and nitric acids as food additives decreased. On the other hand, fresh vegetables and fruits were easily stored in refrigerators and distributed throughout the United States, and the incidence of gastric cancer declined dramatically. Vitamin C in fresh vegetables and fruits acts as an antioxidant and is known to be protective against gastric cancer incidence. Refrigeration was an unexpected triumph against gastric cancer in the United States (Bertuccio et al. 2013).

Nonsteroidal anti-inflammatory drugs and other anti-inflammatory drugs can prevent colon cancer or the formation of polyps (Hamoya et al. 2016). BioBran could also potentially prevent colon cancer and polyp formation, but unfortunately, no clinical study in patients has been conducted to date.

Intestinal flora, food content, and the large intestine's microenvironment are important factors related to colon carcinogenesis. Before the Second World War, colon cancer incidence was relatively rare compared to that of gastric cancer in Japan. Now, the incidence of both cancers is almost the same as those of Western countries. Foods commonly eaten by Japanese people are almost the same as those of developed countries. Foods of fatty content, such as pork, meat, cheese, butter, milk, and eggs, create an oily environment throughout the large intestine with changes to the flora from *Lactobacillus* to anaerobic bacteria such as *Clostridium*. Moreover, the excretory amount of bile must be increased to emulsify and digest the fats by lipase.

Although microinflammation along the entire colon must be almost the same, 75% of colon cancer incidence occurs in the left colon and the rectum (Baran et al. 2018). It occurs because feces of the left colon and rectum are solidified and fractioned to the mucosa with shear stress with modified biliary chemicals such as methylcholanthrene leading to microinflammation in the mucosal wall of the colon, especially the left colon.

9.6 Human Papillomavirus and Cervical Cancer

Carcinogenesis of the uterine cervix is closely related to human papillomavirus (HPV). However, viral integration of the patient genome has not been detected. Almost one in 1000 people who are HPV+ may suffer from cervical cancer. In this case, the local inflammatory process around the cervical area is also promoting carcinogenesis, such as sexual intercourse or a pessary. The pap smear screening test for cervix cancer should be promoted, so is taking anti-inflammatory dietary supplements. Clinical studies using BioBran in this field should be planned. According to a cost-performance analysis and an immunological point of view (Laprise et al. 2020), a HPV vaccine with a low percentage of side effects should be a second choice.

9.7 Hepatocellular Carcinoma

Almost all patients with hepatocellular carcinoma occur in the process of chronic hepatitis. Non-cirrhotic patients with hepatocellular carcinoma are quite rare. Follow-up studies of liver biopsy of patients with liver cirrhosis with hepatitis B virus (HBV) infection and hepatitis C virus (HCV) infection show a close relationship with the grade of inflammation. Viral integration in the patient DNA in the case of HBV remains to be clarified (Nault et al. 2015). Also, viral integration in the patient RNA in the case of HCV remains to be clarified. BioBran has been shown to be useful for the treatment of patients with hepatocellular carcinoma (Bang et al. 2010).

Recently, patients with hepatocellular carcinoma with non-HBV or non-HCV hepatitis increased and were suffering from nonalcoholic fatty liver disease due to obesity with hepatocellular carcinoma. These findings support the notion that chronic inflammatory processes themselves, that is, "friendly-fire," must be closely related to carcinogenesis of the liver (Tateishi et al. 2015). Thus, the theory of viral carcinogenesis and viral integration of carcinogenesis is not correct, but microinflammation in the liver due to any etiology is the fundamental cause of hepatocellular carcinoma.

9.8 Atherosclerosis and Arteriosclerosis

Atherosclerosis occurs along the elastic part of the arterial system, such as the aorta and its main branches, the coronary and carotid arteries. The last two systems are target arteries of ischemic disease due to atheroma formation leading to stenosis or obstruction. Arterioles are the weakest point of ischemic change in every organ, especially in the heart, brain, and kidney, because they are the primary resistance vessels against the pulsatile power of the arterial blood from the heart (Mayet and Hughes 2003). Not only arterial pressure but also cigarette oxidants are initiators of endothelial damage leading to local inflammation.

In the arterial wall, the endothelium of the arterial system is covered along the inner wall of the arteries and arterioles (Lewis et al. 2020). They are always attacked by the pulsatile shear stress of circulation during the heartbeat. If blood pressure is higher than normal, then the endothelium is always enduring higher shear stress, and then it is damaged or degenerated. The endothelia become the center of microinflammation and thrombotic reaction, which is the locus of "friendly-fire" of nonspecific inflammation of eicosanoid pathways by infiltrating macrophages and neutrophils. Therefore, chronically taking aspirin or an anti-inflammatory dietary supplement like BioBran is reasonable to shut down the eicosanoid pathways.

Arteriosclerosis refers to sclerosis or the process of scar formation by an inflammatory process. In the case of hypertension, repeating shear stress must occur by "friendly-fire" in the arterial wall leading to the inflammatory and fibrosing (scarring) processes of arteriosclerosis. Since arterioles throughout the body play the main role in resisting arterial blood pressure, they are called resistance vessels. As the result of arteriolar resistance, the capillary area is not under the pulsatile environment, called the microcirculatory environment. Even mild hypertension for a long period is at risk of causing microinflammation and thrombotic changes in the arterial system. Thus, an anti-inflammatory dietary supplement, such as BioBran, is warranted to prevent the microinflammatory process leading to arteriosclerosis. This inflammatory process of the arterial intima can be monitored by assessing highly sensitive C-reactive protein (CRP) (Pepys et al. 2006).

Recently, lectin-like oxidized low-density lipoprotein receptor and CRP became important to analyze the microinflammation of arteriosclerosis (Fujita et al. 2009). According to all of the evidence, initiating and promoting ischemic disease factors of the heart and brain may be closely related to microinflammation, which BioBran could protect. CRP is a useful biomarker for health screening and checking the immune system's balance (Kaptoge et al. 2010).

9.9 Alzheimer's Disease

β-amyloid and τ proteins are ordinarily metabolized and excreted from the brain by newly discovered lymphatics and then in urine from the body as catabolized nitrogen substances from protein (Aspelund et al. 2015). Those nitrogen catabolites in the brain can be sufficiently washed out through intracerebral lymphatics to the deep cervical lymphatics at a younger age. However, catabolism of τ and then β-amyloid proteins might be genetically or relatively insufficient in excretion capacity which leads to deposits in nerve cells. Finally, the three-dimensional amyloid structure of the β-amyloid protein in nerve cells is called senile plaques. Intraneuronal deposition of τ protein is called neurofibrillary tangles. These changes of nerve cells are supported by astrocytes and phagocytosed by microglia. Then, nerve cells might be necrotized, leading to local microinflammation in the release of arachidonic acid and eicosanoid cascade. Thus, it is reasonable to assume that the anti-inflammatory effect of BioBran could prevent the progress of neurological abnormalities or progression of dementia. BioBran should be further researched in patients with Alzheimer's disease.

9.10 Summary

Three organ systems, the immune, endocrine, and autonomic nervous, are fundamental to our body for daily life and life expectancy. These three systems are closely connected, especially after discovering the acetylcholine receptor on T lymphocytes and macrophages by Mashimo et al. (2019). This former missing link now shows the cross-contact of the three systems, revealing a new view of human life. Moreover, the hypothalamus is the emotional center and the control tower of the endocrine and autonomic nervous systems, and acetylcholine plays a vital role as the molecular link between neurotransmitter and as an immune system cytokine. BioBran can play a crucial role in supporting these three systems.

The immunomodulating and anti-inflammatory effects of BioBran, mentioned above, provide excellent support during inflammatory disease. Moreover, our fundamental health is supported by the hematopoietic immune system. In this regard, Ghoneum et al. have shown that BioBran could protect our hematopoietic immune system (Ghoneum et al. 2013). The functional decline of the hematopoietic system is closely associated with the aging from the anatomopathological point of view. Optimal functioning of the three systems mentioned above and a sound hematopoietic system, supported by BioBran, could give us a sound centenarian life.

References

Ariel IM, Avery EE, Kanter L, Head JR, Langston HT (1950) Primary carcinoma of the lung. A clinical study of 1205 cases. Cancer 3:229–239

Aspelund A, Antila S, Proulx ST, Karlsen TV, Karaman S, Detmar M et al (2015) A dural lymphatic vascular system that drains brain interstitial fluid and macromolecules. J Exp Med 212:991–999

Bang MH, Van Riep T, Thinh NT, Song LH, Dung TT, Van Troung L et al (2010) Arabinoxylan rice bran (MGN-3) enhances the effects of interventional therapies for the treatment of hepatocellular carcinoma: a three-year randomized clinical trial. Anticancer Res 30:5145–5151

Baran B, Mert Ozupek N, Yerli Tetik N, Acar E, Bekcioglu O, Baskin Y (2018) Difference between left-sided and right-sided colorectal cancer: a focused review of literature. Gastroenterol Res 11: 264–273

Bertuccio P, Rosato V, Andreano A, Ferraroni M, Decarli A, Edefonti V et al (2013) Dietary patterns and gastric cancer risk: a systematic review and meta-analysis. Ann Oncol 24:1450–1458

Endo Y (2004) Cancer and inflammation: the potential for prevention. Mag Complement Altern Med Prof 4:32–34

Endo Y, Kanbayashi H (2003) Modified rice bran beneficial for weight loss of mice as a major and acute adverse effect of cisplatin. Pharmacol Toxicol 92:300–303

Endo Y, Kanbayashi H, Hara M (1993) Experimental immunoglobulin A nephropathy induced by gram-negative bacteria. Nephron 65:196–205

Franceschi C, Bonafè M, Valensin S, Olivieri F, De Luca M, Ottaviani E et al (2000) Inflamm-aging. An evolutionary perspective on immunosenescence. Ann N Y Acad Sci 908:244–254
Fujiki H (2014) Gist of Dr. Katsusaburo Yamagiwa's papers entitled "Experimental study on the pathogenesis of epithelial tumors" (I to VI reports). Cancer Sci 105:143–149
Fujita Y, Kakino A, Nishimichi N, Yamaguchi S, Sato Y, Machida S et al (2009) Oxidized LDL receptor LOX-1 binds to C-reactive protein and mediates its vascular effects. Clin Chem 55: 285–294
Gaddy JA, Radin JN, Loh JT, Zhang F, Washington MK, Peek RM Jr et al (2013) High dietary salt intake exacerbates Helicobacter pylori-induced gastric carcinogenesis. Infect Immun 81:2258–2267
Ghoneum M (2016) From bench to bedside : the growing use of arabinoxylan rice bran (MGN-3/Biobran) in cancer immunotherapy. Austin Immunol 1:1006
Ghoneum M, Abedi S (2004) Enhancement of natural killer cell activity of aged mice by modified arabinoxylan rice bran (MGN-3/Biobran). J Pharm Pharmacol 56:1581–1588
Ghoneum M, Badr El-Din NK, Fattah SMA, Tolentino L (2013) Arabinoxylan rice bran (MGN-3/Biobran) provides protection against whole-body γ-irradiation in mice via restoration of hematopoietic tissues. J Radiat Res 54:419
Hamoya T, Fujii G, Miyamoto S, Takahashi M, Totsuka Y, Wakabayashi K et al (2016) Effects of NSAIDs on the risk factors of colorectal cancer: a mini review. Genes Environ 38:6
Hecht SS (2012) Lung carcinogenesis by tobacco smoke. Int J Cancer 131:2724–2732
Hoshino Y, Hirashima N, Nakanishi M, Furuno T (2010) Inhibition of degranulation and cytokine production in bone marrow-derived mast cells by hydrolyzed rice bran. Inflamm Res 59:615–625
Kanbayashi H, Endo Y (2002) Evaluation of the effects of asthma prevention and symptom reduction by enzymatically modified rice-bran foods in asthmatic model mice. Jpn J Allergol 51: 957
Kaptoge S, Di Angelantonio E, Lowe G, Pepys MB, Thompson SG, Collins R et al (2010) C-reactive protein concentration and risk of coronary heart disease, stroke, and mortality: an individual participant meta-analysis. Lancet 375:132–140
Laprise J-F, Chesson HW, Markowitz LE, Drolet M, Martin D, Bénard É et al (2020) Effectiveness and cost-effectiveness of human papillomavirus vaccination through age 45 years in the United States. Ann Intern Med 172:22–29
Lee J, Taneja V, Vassallo R (2012) Cigarette smoking and inflammation: cellular and molecular mechanisms. J Dent Res 91:142–149
Lewis JE, Atlas SE, Abbas MH, Rasul A, Farooqi A, Lantigua LA et al (2020) Cardiovascular, endothelial function, and immune markers in response to treatment with a polysaccharide in HIV(+) adults in a randomized, double-blind placebo-controlled trial. J Clin Transl Res 5:140–147
Liu Y, Chen H, Sun Z, Chen X (2015) Molecular mechanisms of ethanol-associated oro-esophageal squamous cell carcinoma. Cancer Lett 361:164–173
Loomis D, Guyton KZ, Grosse Y, Lauby-Secretan B, El Ghissassi F, Bouvard V et al (2016) Carcinogenicity of drinking coffee, mate, and very hot beverages. Lancet Oncol 17:877–878
Markus J, Miller A, Smith M, Orengo I (2006) Metastatic hemangiopericytoma of the skin treated with wide local excision and MGN-3. Dermatol Surg 32:145–147
Mashimo M, Komori M, Matsui YY, Murase MX, Fujii T, Takeshima S et al (2019) Distinct roles of α7 nAChRs in antigen-presenting cells and CD4(+) T cells in the regulation of T cell differentiation. Front Immunol 10:1102
Mayet J, Hughes A (2003) Cardiac and vascular pathophysiology in hypertension. Heart 89:1104–1109
Musk AW, de Klerk NH (2003) History of tobacco and health. Respirology 8:286–290
Nault J-C, Datta S, Imbeaud S, Franconi A, Mallet M, Couchy G et al (2015) Recurrent AAV2-related insertional mutagenesis in human hepatocellular carcinomas. Nat Genet 47:1187–1193

Ooi SL, McMullen D, Golombick T, Pak SC (2018) Evidence-based review of BioBran/MGN-3 arabinoxylan compound as a complementary therapy for conventional cancer treatment. Integr Cancer Ther 17:165–178

Pepys MB, Hirschfield GM, Tennent GA, Ruth Gallimore J, Kahan MC, Bellotti V et al (2006) Targeting C-reactive protein for the treatment of cardiovascular disease. Nature 440:1217–1221

Seelig MG, Benignus EL (1936) Coal smoke soot and tumors of the lung in mice. Am J Cancer 28: 96–111

Sharan RN, Mehrotra R, Choudhury Y, Asotra K (2012) Association of betel nut with carcinogenesis: revisit with a clinical perspective. PLoS One 7:e42759–e42759

Tateishi R, Okanoue T, Fujiwara N, Okita K, Kiyosawa K, Omata M et al (2015) Clinical characteristics, treatment, and prognosis of non-B, non-C hepatocellular carcinoma: a large retrospective multicenter cohort study. J Gastroenterol 50:350–360

Wang X-Q, Terry P-D, Yan H (2009) Review of salt consumption and stomach cancer risk: epidemiological and biological evidence. World J Gastroenterol 15:2204–2213

Zielen S, Bröker M, Strnad N, Schwenen L, Schön P, Gottwald G et al (1996) Simple determination of polysaccharide specific antibodies by means of chemically modified ELISA plates. J Immunol Methods 193:1–7

Human Immunodeficiency Virus (HIV) 10

Sok Cheon Pak, Soo Liang Ooi, Peter S. Micalos, Kentaro Ninomiya, and Mamdooh H. Ghoneum

Abstract

Acquired immune deficiency syndrome (AIDS) is the most advanced stage of human immunodeficiency virus (HIV) infection. As a retrovirus, HIV-1 is more virulent and prevalent compared to HIV-2. HIV infection leads to progressive loss of CD4+ T cells. The depletion of CD4+ T cells triggers a wide range of immunological abnormalities and hematological changes, increasing the risk of opportunistic infections and malignancies due to immunodeficiency. The current regimen of antiretroviral treatment (ART) is not curative, but durable viral load suppression is continued so that the person with HIV can maintain high CD4+ T cells for sustainable living. Although ART extends life expectancy, there comes a point where immunomodulation aiming to reduce HIV-associated immune activation and enhance the immune response to control HIV infection is still required. Biobran is a potent biological response modifier with immunomodulatory properties. The potential anti-HIV activity of Biobran was demonstrated via augmentation of lymphocyte proliferation in an HIV-infected individual. Biobran supplementation could potentially improve CD4+ T cells and CD4/CD8 ratio in HIV positive patients. Such findings support the potential use of Biobran as an adjunct therapy for people living with HIV.

S. C. Pak (✉) · S. L. Ooi · P. S. Micalos
School of Dentistry and Medical Sciences, Charles Sturt University, Bathurst, NSW, Australia
e-mail: spak@csu.edu.au

K. Ninomiya
Daiwa Pharmaceutical Co., Ltd., Tokyo, Japan

M. H. Ghoneum
Department of Surgery, Charles R. Drew University of Medicine and Science, Los Angeles, CA, USA

S. C. Pak et al. (eds.), *Modified Rice Bran Arabinoxylan*,
https://doi.org/10.1007/978-981-19-5735-2_10

Keywords

AIDS · HIV · CD4+ T cells · Immunomodulation · Biobran

10.1 Introduction

The prevalence of human immunodeficiency virus/acquired immune deficiency syndrome (HIV/AIDS) continues to be a major challenge to public health authorities worldwide. In 2020 an estimated 38 million people lived with HIV (including 1.7 million children), with a global prevalence of 0.7% among adults (UNAIDS 2021). Given the severity of the current pandemic, it is not surprising that the dynamic of COVID-19 has widened existing inequalities, which block progress to ending AIDS. The Joint United Nations Programme on HIV/AIDS (UNAIDS) Coordinating Board has adopted a Global AIDS Strategy 2012–2026 to recommend every country to end AIDS as a public health threat by 2030 (UNAIDS Board adopts new global AIDS strategy which paves the way to end AIDS by 2030 2021). The Global AIDS Strategy puts people at the center and aims to unite all communities to take prioritized action to transform health and life outcomes for people living with and affected by HIV.

HIV is a retrovirus consisting of an envelope protein containing two identical single-stranded RNA molecules (German Advisory Committee Blood (Arbeitskreis Blut) and Subgroup 'Assessment of Pathogens Transmissible by Blood' 2016). There are two main types of HIV. HIV-1 is virulent and prevalent, causing the global pandemic. HIV-2 is less pathogenic and is found mainly in West Africa (Esbjörnsson et al. 2019). The more aggressive HIV-1 can be transmitted through body fluids from infected persons, such as blood, breast milk, semen, or vaginal secretions. Unprotected sexual intercourse and sharing of percutaneous inoculation equipment are the typical transmission modes (Shaw and Hunter 2012). Without antiretroviral treatment (ART), there is also a high risk of mother-to-child transmission during gestation, labor, and breastfeeding (Teasdale et al. 2011).

HIV infection can lead to progressive loss of cluster of differentiation (CD) 4+ T cells, also known as the helper T cells, which play a vital role in the adaptive immune response as they stimulate other lymphocytes to fight infection. The depletion of CD4+ T cells can trigger a wide range of immunological abnormalities and hematological changes, increasing the risks of opportunistic infections and malignancies due to immunodeficiency (Deeks et al. 2015). AIDS is the final stage of HIV infection when the CD4+ T cell count (or CD4 count for short) drops below 200 cells/μl or when there is the presence of any AIDS-defining conditions. HIV infection can be fatal if left untreated, with 8–10 years of median survival time (Sabin 2013).

No cure or vaccine has been found in the 40 years since 1981 when the disease was first reported, even though much progress has been made. The current standard care for HIV infection is a daily ART regimen consisting of two or three HIV medications from different classes. The treatment goal with ART is not curative but durable viral suppression so that the person with HIV can sustain a high CD4 count (>500 cells/μl) and maintain a normal lifespan (Saag et al. 2020). Notwithstanding, ART has not yet fully restored life expectancy to a level comparable to the HIV-free population. Even with successful long-term treatment, people living with HIV are still three times more likely to die than the seronegative cohorts (de Coninck et al. 2018). Hence the search for treatments that can achieve long-term HIV remission is ongoing. Immunomodulation is a promising approach that aims to reduce HIV-associated immune activation and boost immune responses to control HIV infection (Pino et al. 2018).

Biobran, also known as MGN-3 or RBAC, is a modified arabinoxylan compound derived from partially hydrolyzing rice bran using shiitake mushroom enzymes (Ghoneum 1998a). It is a potent biological response modifier with immunomodulatory properties that include upregulating natural killer cell activity (Ghoneum 1998b), augmenting phagocytic cellular functions, modulating cytokine production, promoting T and B lymphocyte proliferation (Ghoneum 1998a), and acting as a natural adjuvant for dendritic cells (Ghoneum and Agrawal 2011). The therapeutic properties of Biobran also include antioxidant, antiangiogenesis, antiproliferative, and anti-inflammatory effects (Ooi et al. 2021). A small amount of research on the effectiveness of Biobran on HIV has been conducted in the view of obtaining clues that could ultimately lead to sustainable usage of Biobran. In this context, this chapter describes a few causal factors for the pathogenicity of HIV infection and how they are affected by Biobran.

10.2 From Infection to CD4+ T Cell Destruction

Once entering the body, HIV will infect the immune cells by attaching and fusing with the host cell membrane, releasing its RNA strands in the process. Through reverse transcription, the injected RNA is converted into proviral DNA and carried into the cell nucleus, where it binds to and is integrated with the host DNA. The host cell is compromised at this stage, and it can be activated to produce copies of HIV particles to infect other cells (German Advisory Committee Blood (Arbeitskreis Blut) and Subgroup 'Assessment of Pathogens Transmissible by Blood' 2016). The infection will spread through the lymphoid system starting from the mucosal tissues. The HIV RNA will become detectable in the blood becoming viremia after a few days. Viral load will increase exponentially until its peak in a few weeks associated with a transient reduction in peripheral CD4+ T cells, during which the adaptive immune response is triggered to release antibodies against HIV (Deeks et al. 2015). These events signify the acute phase of HIV infection, and some patients may experience nonspecific symptoms such as fever, fatigue, muscle pain, headache, and swollen lymph nodes, collectively known as acute retroviral syndrome (ARS) (Crowell et al. 2018). Patients with ARS have a higher viral burden and lower CD4 count, and they experience immune activation across multiple body compartments compared to those without ARS (Crowell et al. 2018). The host antibodies against the HIV viral particles can only achieve partial control in reducing the viral load without eliminating the infectious agents (Baum 2010).

Not all CD4+ T cells are equal as HIV preferentially infects a subset called HIV-specific CD4+ T cells. A study performed on 12 HIV-infected individuals showed that HIV-specific memory CD4+ T cells in infected individuals contained more HIV viral DNA than other memory CD4+ T cells at all stages of HIV disease (Douek et al. 2002). Additionally, following viral rebound during interruption of ART, the frequency of HIV viral DNA in the HIV-specific pool of memory CD4+ T cells increased to a greater extent than in memory CD4+ T cells of other specificities. Nevertheless, HIV-specific CD4+ T cells do play a protective role towards viremia and disease progression. For the rare individuals who can control HIV replication after infection without ART, called elite controllers, their HIV-specific CD4+ T cells showed higher avidity than patients with progressive infection (Chevalier et al. 2016; Porichis and Kaufmann 2011). HIV-specific CD4+ T cell dysfunction results from altered differentiation that leads to disease progression (Morou et al. 2019).

The disease becomes chronic after 4–6 months with the establishment of a steady-state viremia level or set-point. The set-point is highly variable across individuals, ranging from 1000 to 1 million viral copies per milliliter (Fraser et al. 2007). Naturally, those with higher set-points are more likely to have immune dysfunction, high levels of inflammation, and higher risk of rapid disease progression (Deeks et al. 2015). Nonetheless, a rebound of CD4 count from the low level during the acute phase can be observed in all patients. Patients will continue to experience progressive loss of CD4+ T cells through destruction and decreased production. Eventually, it will lead to AIDS if left untreated. Thus, the depletion of CD4+ T cells is a hallmark of AIDS, and the CD4 count is a commonly used marker of HIV disease progression.

With the success of modern ART in suppressing HIV, many patients still succumb to non-AIDS–defining conditions, such as cardiovascular disease, liver disease, kidney disease, malignancies, and others due to persistent immune dysfunction despite normalization of CD4 count (McBride and Striker 2017). Therefore, CD4 count and viral load are no longer sufficient to estimate the risks facing HIV patients. The role of CD8+ T cells in HIV disease progression has become increasingly prominent. Being the cytotoxic effector cells that directly destroy virus-infected cells, CD8+ T cells are essential in controlling HIV replication during the acute stage of the infection. However, their cytotoxic potential decreases dramatically with disease progression, leading to a diminishing capacity to exert antiviral response (Perdomo-Celis et al. 2019). The CD8+ T cells suffer immune exhaustion, altering their profile and becoming progressively dysfunctional. The number of dysfunctional CD8+ T cells continues to increase in chronic HIV infection (Perdomo-Celis et al. 2019). Hence, the balance between CD4+ T cells and CD8+ T cells (or CD4/CD8 ratio) has been suggested as a more reliable prognostic marker for the HIV-positive population (McBride and Striker 2017). A normal CD4/CD8 ratio is greater than 1.0, and most HIV-infected individuals with long-term viral suppression still had a persistent inversion of CD4/CD8 ratio (<1) (Caby et al. 2016). Naturally, low CD4/CD8 ratio and high CD8+ T cell count were associated with non-AIDS–defining conditions and excess AIDS mortality in an HIV population (Perdomo-Celis et al. 2019; Gojak et al. 2019).

10.3 The Potential Benefits of Biobran Against HIV

10.3.1 In Vitro Anti-HIV Effects

Ghoneum showed that Biobran possesses anti-HIV potential in two in vitro experiments (Ghoneum 1998a). First, mononuclear cells (MNCs) were isolated from the human peripheral blood of three healthy volunteers and cultured with the HIV-1 SF strain. Infected MNCs were incubated with Biobran at various concentrations (0–100 μg/ml) for 7 days at 37 °C. The culture supernatants of HIV-1 infected cells were collected at the end of the incubation period for viral production analysis using the HIV-1 p24 ELISA kit. The results showed that Biobran inhibited HIV viral replication in a dose-dependent manner. Biobran treatment at concentrations of 12.5, 25, 50, and 100 μg/ml inhibited HIV-1 p24 antigen production by 18.3, 42.8, 59, and 75%, respectively, relative to viral production without Biobran (Ghoneum 1998a).

Syncytia, the multinucleated cell products from cell fusion, are associated with AIDS and represent a "danger" signal capable of triggering inflammatory responses (Compton and Schwartz 2017). Another in vitro experiment by Ghoneum studied the effect of Biobran on HIV-induced syncytia formation (Ghoneum 1998a). Again, peripheral blood MNCs from five AIDS patients were cultured at 37 °C in the presence of Biobran at various concentrations (0–100 μg/ml). The cultures were examined after 7 days with the total number of syncytia counted. Results showed that Biobran inhibited the number of syncytia formation in a dose-dependent manner with a 38.5, 50, 62.5, and 75% reduction for Biobran concentrations of 12.5, 25, 50, and 100 μg/ml, respectively (Ghoneum 1998a). These two pre-clinical experiments clearly demonstrated that Biobran possesses an inhibitory effect on HIV replication in vitro, and they formed the basis of all subsequent human studies on the potential use of Biobran as an adjunct therapy for HIV.

10.3.2 Lymphocyte Proliferation

Lymphocyte proliferation is a fundamental characteristic of the host immune system in response to antigenic stimulation. In untreated HIV infection, both CD4+ and CD8+ T cells significantly increased compared to the levels observed in healthy individuals. Such peripheral T cell proliferation results from generalized immune activation (Hazenberg et al. 2000). A recent study has reported that the CD4+ T cell proliferation level during acute HIV-1 infection was inversely correlated with the decline of CD4+ T cells 2 years later. Hence, CD4+ T cell proliferation is effective in the acute phase and is beneficial to preserving CD4 cell count subsequently (Xia et al. 2018).

The in vivo effect of Biobran on lymphocyte proliferation was studied by Ghoneum in human subjects. Five healthy volunteers were given Biobran at 15 mg/kg/day orally for 2 months. MNCs were prepared from the peripheral blood of these individuals. Significant increases in T and B cell mitogen responses after Biobran treatment were observed compared to the values at baseline, suggesting the augmentory effect of Biobran on lymphocyte proliferation (Ghoneum 1998a). Thus, the immunomodulatory effects of Biobran could potentially promote T cell proliferation during acute HIV infection and possibly sustain CD4 cell count and CD4/CD8 balance among HIV+ individuals in the longer term.

10.3.3 CD4+ T Cell Count and CD4/CD8 Ratio

The positive effect of Biobran on the CD4+ T cell recovery trend was reported in a case study of a 22-year-old male with known anti-HIV seropositive status (Chaiyasit and Wiwanitkit 2020). The patient had denied ART and started taking Biobran (4 g/day) with no other concomitant treatment. After 1 month, his CD4 cell count increased 1.4-fold from baseline (499 cells/μl to 715 cells/μl), and his CD4+ T cell percentage increased from 27.88% to 34%.

This finding was further supported by a recent clinical trial (Lewis et al. 2020) wherein 22 HIV-infected patients on stable ART were assigned to the Biobran group for 6 months. When analyzed for CD4+ T cell count, Biobran (3 g/day) caused a modest (nonsignificant) short-term (3 months) improvement compared to their baseline value. Compared to another 25 HIV patients on ART and placebo, the study found a statistically significant ($p = 0.04$) percentage change in the CD8+ T cell count between the two groups. At the end of 6 months, the Biobran group showed a 5.2% decrease, whereas the placebo group's value increased by 57.8%. Notably, the CD4/CD8 ratio increased in the Biobran group (0.95 ± 0.62 to 1.07 ± 0.7) but decreased in the placebo group (0.96 ± 0.8 to 0.72 ± 0.59). Even though the change was statistically marginal ($p = 0.085$) between groups, it was considered clinically significant for the Biobran group to reach CD4/CD8 ratio normalization (Lewis et al. 2020).

10.3.4 Systolic Blood Pressure and Endothelial Function

Patients with HIV on ART suffer from hypertension and endothelial dysfunction; however, conventional treatment does not alleviate such issues. Recent evidence indicates that the increased cardiovascular risk in HIV-infected individuals is attributable to HIV infection itself (Anand et al. 2018). HIV as a retrovirus can produce the envelope glycoproteins such as gp120, Tat, and Nef. These viral proteins play a major role in the pathogenesis of endothelial dysfunction, which is a precursor of cardiovascular events, including atherosclerosis (Anand et al. 2018).

In the randomized, double-blind placebo-controlled trial, Biobran was reported to positively affect the systolic blood pressure and endothelial function of HIV+

patients on stable ART (Lewis et al. 2020). Systolic blood pressure as a cardiovascular marker decreased in the Biobran group, while it increased in the placebo group. However, there was no clear trend in the skin blood flow in response to nitric oxide as an endothelial function marker between groups. Further analysis using multivariate repeated measures analysis of variance model revealed that treatment effect (Biobran vs. placebo) was significant ($p < 0.001$) for the systolic blood pressure and endothelial function over time. Thus, Biobran treatment may improve the overall health profile of HIV+ individuals through modest short-term improvements in their cardiovascular biomarkers.

10.4 Conclusion

Research into the medical application of Biobran to treat HIV is limited despite its growing use in cancer immunotherapy. This chapter highlights the key players of HIV disease progression and their modification following Biobran administration. The potential anti-HIV activity of Biobran was demonstrated via inhibition of HIV-1 replication and syncytia formation in vitro. Furthermore, augmented lymphocyte proliferation by Biobran was shown in healthy subjects and an HIV+ patient case study. Biobran supplementation could potentially improve CD4 count and CD4/CD8 ratio in HIV-infected patients, suggesting T cell homeostasis through the suppression of specific T cell responses to immunopathology. Finally, Biobran was shown to improve systolic blood pressure and endothelial function in HIV-infected individuals. Further research is needed to explore the potential use of Biobran as an adjunct therapy to enhance the immune and health profile of people living with HIV.

References

Anand AR, Rachel G, Parthasarathy D (2018) HIV proteins and endothelial dysfunction: implications in cardiovascular disease. Front Cardiovasc Med 5:185

Baum LL (2010) Role of humoral immunity in host defense against HIV. Curr HIV/AIDS Rep 7: 11–18

Caby F, Guihot A, Lambert-Niclot S, Guiguet M, Boutolleau D, Agher R et al (2016) Determinants of a low CD4/CD8 ratio in HIV-1–infected individuals despite long-term viral suppression. Clin Infect Dis 62:1297–1303

Chaiyasit K, Wiwanitkit V (2020) CD4+ count after arabinoxylan supplementation: an observation. Indian J Sex Transm Dis AIDS 41:129

Chevalier MF, Didier C, Girard P-M, Manea ME, Campa P, Barré-Sinoussi F et al (2016) CD4 T-cell responses in primary HIV infection: interrelationship with immune activation and virus burden. Front Immunol 7:395

Compton AA, Schwartz O (2017) They might be giants: does syncytium formation sink or spread HIV infection? PLoS Pathog 13:e1006099

Crowell TA, Colby DJ, Pinyakorn S, Fletcher JLK, Kroon E, Schuetz A et al (2018) Acute retroviral syndrome is associated with high viral burden, CD4 depletion, and immune activation in systemic and tissue compartments. Clin Infect Dis 66:1540–1549 de Coninck Z, Hussain-Alkhateeb L, Bratt G, Ekström AM, Gisslén M, Petzold M et al (2018) Non-AIDS mortality is higher among successfully treated people living with HIV compared with matched HIV-negative control persons: a 15-year follow-up cohort study in Sweden. AIDS Patient Care STDs 32:297–305

Deeks SG, Overbaugh J, Phillips A, Buchbinder S (2015) HIV infection. Nat Rev Dis Prim 1:15035

Douek DC, Brenchley JM, Betts MR, Ambrozak DR, Hill BJ, Okamoto Y et al (2002) HIV preferentially infects HIV-specific CD4+ T cells. Nature 417:95–98

Esbjörnsson J, Jansson M, Jespersen S, Månsson F, Hønge BL, Lindman J et al (2019) HIV-2 as a model to identify a functional HIV cure. AIDS Res Ther 16:24

Fraser C, Hollingsworth TD, Chapman R, de Wolf F, Hanage WP (2007) Variation in HIV-1 set-point viral load: epidemiological analysis and an evolutionary hypothesis. Proc Natl Acad Sci 104:17441–17446

German Advisory Committee Blood (Arbeitskreis Blut), Subgroup 'Assessment of Pathogens Transmissible by Blood' (2016) Human Immunodeficiency Virus (HIV). Transfus Med Hemother 43:203–222

Ghoneum M (1998a) Anti-HIV activity in vitro of MGN-3, an activated arabinoxylane from rice bran. Biochem Biophys Res Commun 243:25–29

Ghoneum M (1998b) Enhancement of human natural killer cell activity by modified arabinoxylane from rice bran (MGN-3). Int J Immunother 14:89–99

Ghoneum M, Agrawal S (2011) Activation of human monocyte-derived dendritic cells in vitro by biological response modifier arabinoxylan rice bran (MGN-3/Biobran). Int J Immunopathol Pharmacol 24:941–948

Gojak R, Hadžiosmanović V, Baljić R, Zečević L, Ćorić J, Mijailović Ž (2019) CD4/CD8 ratio as a predictor for the occurrence of metabolic syndrome in HIV/AIDS patients during 6 months of cART therapy. J Med Biochem 38:489–495

Hazenberg MD, Stuart JWTC, Otto SA, Borleffs JCC, Boucher CAB, de Boer RJ et al (2000) T-cell division in human immunodeficiency virus (HIV)-1 infection is mainly due to immune activation: a longitudinal analysis in patients before and during highly active antiretroviral therapy (HAART). Blood 95:249–255

Lewis JE, Atlas SE, Abbas MH, Rasul A, Farooqi A, Lantigua LA et al (2020) Cardiovascular, endothelial function, and immune markers in response to treatment with a polysaccharide in HIV(+) adults in a randomized, double-blind placebo-controlled trial. J Clin Transl Res 5:140–147

McBride JA, Striker R (2017) Imbalance in the game of T cells: what can the CD4/CD8 T-cell ratio tell us about HIV and health? PLoS Pathog 13:e1006624

Morou A, Brunet-Ratnasingham E, Dubé M, Charlebois R, Mercier E, Darko S et al (2019) Altered differentiation is central to HIV-specific CD4+ T cell dysfunction in progressive disease. Nat Immunol 20:1059–1070

Ooi SL, Pak SC, Micalos PS, Schupfer E, Lockley C, Park MH et al (2021) The health-promoting properties and clinical applications of rice bran arabinoxylan modified with shiitake mushroom enzyme—a narrative review. Molecules 26:2539

Perdomo-Celis F, Taborda NA, Rugeles MT (2019) CD8+ T-cell response to HIV infection in the era of antiretroviral therapy. Front Immunol 10:1896

Pino M, Paiardini M, Marconi VC (2018) Progress in achieving long-term HIV remission. Curr Opin HIV AIDS 13:435–445

Porichis F, Kaufmann DE (2011) HIV-specific CD4 T cells and immune control of viral replication. Curr Opin HIV AIDS 6:174–180

Saag MS, Gandhi RT, Hoy JF, Landovitz RJ, Thompson MA, Sax PE et al (2020) Antiretroviral drugs for treatment and prevention of HIV infection in adults: 2020 recommendations of the International Antiviral Society–USA panel. JAMA 324:1651–1669

Sabin CA (2013) Do people with HIV infection have a normal life expectancy in the era of combination antiretroviral therapy? BMC Med 11:251

Shaw GM, Hunter E (2012) HIV transmission. Cold Spring Harb Perspect Med 2:a006965

Teasdale CA, Marais BJ, Abrams EJ (2011) HIV: prevention of mother-to-child transmission. BMJ Clin Evid 2011:909

UNAIDS (2021) Global HIV & AIDS statistics — Fact sheet [Internet]. https://www.unaids.org/en/resources/fact-sheet

UNAIDS Board adopts new global AIDS strategy which paves the way to end AIDS by 2030 (2021) UNAIDS press release [internet]. Geneva, Switzerland. https://www.unaids.org/en/resources/presscentre/pressreleaseandstatementarchive/2021/march/20210325_new-global-aids-strategy

Xia H, Jiang W, Zhang X, Qin L, Su B, Li Z et al (2018) Elevated level of CD4(+) T cell immune activation in acutely HIV-1-infected stage associates with increased IL-2 production and cycling expression, and subsequent CD4(+) T cell preservation. Front Immunol 9:616

Hepatitis

11

Yukari Egashira

Abstract

This chapter introduces the effects of arabinoxylan rice bran (Biobran) on hepatitis in animals and humans based on evidence-based research papers. The liver plays an important role in a variety of physiological functions. Liver damage can develop with diseases such as hepatitis and nonalcoholic fatty liver disease (NAFLD). Hepatitis induced by D-galactosamine is a well-studied animal research model that is histologically and pathologically similar to the effects of human hepatitis B virus. Supplementation with Biobran suppressed the D-galactosamine-induced hepatitis and IL-18 expression in rats by inhibition of NF-kappaB and JNK/MAPK expression. Moreover, Biobran supplementation (1 g/day, 3 months) showed suppressed viremia levels in patients infected with chronic hepatitis C virus. In patients with NAFLD, Biobran was consumed 1 g/day for 90 days. The level of alkaline phosphatase significantly decreased in the Biobran feeding group compared to placebo ($p < 0.05$). More clinical and basic research on Biobran is required in the future to clarify its supportive effects and mechanisms of action in hepatitis.

Keywords

Arabinoxylan rice bran (Biobran) · Interleukin-18 · Nonalcoholic fatty liver disease · Hepatitis C virus · D-Galactosamine-induced hepatitis

Y. Egashira (✉)
Laboratory of Food and Nutrition, Division of Applied Biochemistry, Graduate School of Horticulture, Chiba University, Matsudo, Chiba, Japan
e-mail: egashira@faculty.chiba-u.jp

S. C. Pak et al. (eds.), *Modified Rice Bran Arabinoxylan*,
https://doi.org/10.1007/978-981-19-5735-2_11

11.1 Hepatitis

The liver plays an important role in a variety of physiological functions, including metabolism, xenobiotic detoxification, storage, and secretion. Therefore, when the liver is damaged, it can cause a variety of metabolic disorders and diseases such as hepatitis, fatty liver, and nonalcoholic fatty liver disease (NAFLD).

Hepatitis has become a global health problem that is associated with significant morbidity and mortality. Therefore, it is important to prevent or treat hepatitis with medications or other treatments. In humans, hepatitis is often caused by viruses, drugs, or alcohol. In animal experiments, D-galactosamine (D-GalN) hepatitis, D-GalN+lipopolysaccharide (LPS)-induced hepatitis, acetaminophen-induced hepatitis, and carbon tetrachloride-induced hepatitis are used as models of acute liver injury. Hepatitis induced by D-GalN is a well-studied model that is histologically and pathophysiologically similar to viral human hepatitis B (Keppler et al. 1968; Decker and Keppler 1974).

11.2 D-GalN Hepatitis (Animal Model) and Arabinoxylan Rice Bran (Biobran)

D-GalN is also found in small amounts in ordinary foods as a component of glycans such as glycoproteins. It has been reported that ingesting a large amount of D-GalN at one time rapidly consumes uridine triphosphate (UTP) when D-GalN is metabolized in the liver (Keppler et al. 1968, 1970; Decker and Keppler 1974). D-GalN hepatitis is thought to be caused by the inhibition of protein and messenger ribonucleic acid (mRNA) biosynthesis due to the depletion of intracellular UTP and enhanced absorption of endotoxin from the intestines to the bloodstream (Galanos et al. 1979; Stachlewitz et al. 1999).

D-GalN administration is known to cause a large increase (i.e., an increase by thousands of times) in the susceptibility to endotoxin. Endotoxin stimulates Kupffer cells in the liver causing tumor necrosis factor-mediated destruction of hepatocytes that results in infiltration of neutrophils and other cells and further hepatocyte necrosis through generation and release of reactive oxygen species (Stachlewitz et al. 1999). Hepatocytes are then destroyed, and activities of the serum hepatic biomarkers alanine transaminase (ALT) and aspartate transaminase (AST) increase. After D-GalN administration, these serum transaminase activity levels reach a maximum at about 24 h and then gradually begin to recover. The D-GalN hepatitis model in rats is not difficult to establish and resembles a certain type of human hepatitis. Therefore, the D-GalN hepatitis model is often used as a model of acute liver injury.

Arabinoxylan rice bran (Biobran, RBAC, or MGN-3) is a modified hemicellulose that can be obtained through partial hydrolysis by enzymes from shiitake mushrooms. Biobran has been reported to have immunomodulatory effects such as activation of natural killer (NK) cells (Ghoneum and Abedi 2004). We investigated the effect of Biobran on the development of D-GalN hepatitis.

Our previous study showed that intake of certain oligosaccharides suppresses D-GalN hepatitis in rats (Wang et al. 1995). Moreover, dietary corn bran hemicellulose (CBH) has been shown to reduce the increase in plasma transaminase activity in D-GalN-treated rats (Daizo et al. 2005, 2006). CBH mainly consists of arabinoxylan. Arabinoxylan hemicellulose is an indigestible polysaccharide that is abundant in cereals such as rice bran or wheat bran. Biobran also suppressed the development of hepatic injury by D-GalN in rats (Zheng et al. 2012a). The serum transaminase (AST and ALT) activity in rats treated with Biobran 1 h before the D-GalN injection was significantly suppressed by both oral administration and intraperitoneal (i.p.) injection. Biobran (20 mg/kg body weight [BW]) was administered i.p., and D-GalN was injected 1 h after the Biobran treatment of the rats. Twenty-four hours after D-GalN treatment, serum samples were collected. AST and ALT activity in the Biobran-treated group was significantly lower than that of the non-Biobran-treated control group (Zheng et al. 2012a). The transaminase values were as follows (mean ± standard error [SE]): AST: control, 1074 ± 76 IU/L and Biobran, 197 ± 7 IU/L; and ALT: control, 239 ± 35 IU/L and Biobran, 14.1 ± 0.7 IU/L. However, at lower Biobran treatment levels, e.g., 0.5 and 5 mg/kg BW, no significant inhibitory effect was observed, while feeding over 30 mg/kg of BW/day of Biobran increased the NK cell activity. A preliminary experiment showed that a large amount of Biobran did not protect against D-GalN hepatitis. Thus, selecting the optimal amount of Biobran is important because of its anti-inflammatory effect.

Next, we hydrolyzed Biobran at 100 °C for 1 h with 1 N HCl to study the active fractions. Following this, the Biobran hydrolysate was neutralized with 1 N NaOH. The solutions were passed through cation and anion resin columns, and the effluent was used in the experiments. Even after this procedure, D-GalN hepatitis was significantly suppressed by Biobran hydrolysate compared with the control (only D-GalN treatment) group (Zheng et al. 2012a). This result indicates that the active components of Biobran are stable despite heating and hydrochloric acid treatment.

We then fractionated Biobran hydrolysate into the following three molecular weights using gel filtration: low, medium, and high. The Biobran hydrolysate and three fractionated materials were administered i.p. Rats in the control group were injected with the same amount of saline. All the groups of mice were injected with D-GalN (400 mg/kg BW) 1 h after treatment with these fractionated Biobran samples (see Reference (Zheng et al. 2012a) for detailed experimental procedures). Hydrolyzed Biobran significantly inhibited D-GalN hepatitis compared with the control, but high molecular weight fractions (≥2,000,000 Da) of Biobran did not inhibit D-GalN hepatitis. Medium molecular weight (400–2,000,000 Da) and low molecular weight (≤400 Da) fractions of Biobran significantly inhibited D-GalN hepatitis in rats. The D-GalN hepatitis inhibitory effect of the low molecular weight Biobran fraction was the strongest among all groups. The transaminase AST values were as follows (mean ± SE): control, 1878 ± 626 IU/L and low molecular weight Biobran fractions, 185 ± 29 IU/L; and ALT: control, 537 ± 261 IU/L and low molecular weight Biobran fractions, 77.8 ± 8.8 IU/L ($p < 0.05$) (Zheng et al. 2012a). The molecular weight of the low molecular weight Biobran fraction was measured using electrospray ionization mass spectrometer (ESIMS), and there was an intense peak at $m/z = 409$. The low molecular weight Biobran fraction was considered to contain oligosaccharide compounds on the basis of the ESIMS results.

The low molecular weight Biobran fraction is a mixture of monosaccharide and oligosaccharides, and glucose is a main component (22.8%). We have reported that several indigestible oligosaccharides such as galacto-oligosaccharide and raffinose inhibit D-GalN hepatitis in rats (Wang et al. 1998). Indigestible oligosaccharides containing galactose had an inhibitory effect on the onset of D-GalN hepatitis. D-GalN hepatitis-suppressive effects of the indigestible oligosaccharides such as raffinose or galacto-oligosaccharide are mediated by intestinal bacteria because raffinose and galacto-oligosaccharide did not inhibit D-GalN hepatitis in rats that were treated with the antibiotic neomycin (Wang et al. 1998). Low molecular weight Biobran fractions contain only a small amount of galactose (0.5%), and thus, it is possible that components different from these galactose-containing oligosaccharides are involved in the suppression of D-GalN hepatitis.

Arabinoxylan hemicellulose is an indigestible polysaccharide that is abundant in cereals that are consumed by humans. Because the chemical bonds between arabinose and xylose and the ratio of arabinose to xylose vary depending on the type of plant, arabinoxylan hemicellulose is thought to have different effects on the liver. In our previous study, we investigated the effect of corn bran hemicellulose (CBH) on D-GalN hepatitis in rats (Daizo et al. 2005, 2006). CBH mainly consists of water-soluble arabinoxylan hemicellulose. CBH also suppressed D-GalN hepatitis. This suppressive effect was observed 7 days after CBH ingestion but not after 1 or 3 days (Daizo et al. 2005). This effect of CBH and other dietary fibers may be related to changes in gut bacteria. However, Biobran suppresses D-GalN hepatitis even after a single dose which suggests that the mechanism is different from that of CBH. In addition, Biobran has been reported to have antioxidant properties (Noaman et al. 2008). Therefore, it is possible that this antioxidant capacity may be related to the prevention of D-GalN-induced hepatitis.

Interleukin (IL)-18 is an inflammatory cytokine that belongs to the IL-1 family. IL-18 is clinically associated with viral liver cirrhosis, primary biliary cirrhosis, or fulminant hepatitis. Serum IL-18 level correlates with the disease severity in patients with these diseases (Tsutsui et al. 2000, 2003). Plasma IL-18 was significantly increased in patients with liver injury that is caused by the hepatitis C virus (HCV) (Murata et al. 2005; Vecchiet et al. 2005). IL-18 is involved in a variety of immunological and inflammatory events (Tsutsui et al. 2000). Finotto et al. reported that IL-18 overexpression has caused substantial hepatitis in mice (Finotto et al. 2004). It was reported that D-GalN hepatitis induced IL-18 in rats and that L-glutamine intake ameliorated the increase of serum IL-18 (Komano et al. 2008). Lu et al. reported that acetaminophen-induced liver injury also caused an increase in IL-18 in mice (Lu et al. 2010). Biobran (20 mg/kg BW, i.p.) and the low molecular weight Biobran fraction (0.5 mg/kg BW, i.p.) administration suppressed IL-18 mRNA expression in the liver and serum IL-18 levels in D-GalN liver injury rats (Zheng et al. 2012a). The hepatoprotective mechanisms were partly mediated by IL-18 downregulation in rats that were administered Biobran.

11.3 Acetaminophen-Induced Hepatitis

We also investigated the effect of Biobran on acetaminophen-induced liver injury in rats. Biobran inhibited the development of acetaminophen hepatotoxicity in rats (Sanada and Egashira 2009). Acetaminophen hepatotoxicity is thought to occur when an intermediate metabolite of acetaminophen is produced by an enzyme in the drug metabolism system, and it binds to reduced glutathione or an enzyme protein thiol group, resulting in abnormal hepatocyte metabolism and ultimately hepatocyte necrosis (Mitchell et al. 1973). D-GalN hepatotoxicity and acetaminophen hepatotoxicity cause hepatitis via different mechanisms. However, Biobran had an inhibitory effect on both types of liver injury in rats. It may act on hepatocyte necrosis and cytotoxicity through neutrophils and other cells, which are common in these two liver disorders.

11.4 Mechanisms of Action

Because IL-18 is involved in the D-GalN hepatitis inhibitory effect of Biobran, we next examined the effect of Biobran on nuclear factor-κB (NF-κB), mitogen-activated protein kinase (MAPK), and CD14 to investigate this mechanism. IL-18 belongs to a novel family of inflammatory cytokines that are related to many kinds of inflammatory and immunological events (Tsutsui et al. 2000). IL-18 is released from murine macrophages or Kupffer cells through the Toll-like receptor 4 (TLR4)/CD14-dependent signaling pathway in animal models (Tsutsui et al. 2003). Activated TLR4/CD14 is associated with alcoholic liver disease and hepatic ischemia (Schwabe et al. 2006; Akira and Hemmi 2003; Peng et al. 2004). TLR4 is a transmembrane protein that is mainly present in macrophages. TLR4 recognizes LPS, which is a constitutive element of the bacterial cell wall, or the LPS/CD14 complex, and it mediates macrophage activation and pro-inflammatory cytokine production and release (Peng et al. 2004). CD14 is a key gene in the innate immune system and functions as a LPS receptor. CD14/LPS interactions at the level of the membrane activate TLR-4, which plays an important role in signal transduction in the innate immune response (Peng et al. 2004). It is well known that TLR4 activates a transcription factor, NF-κB, and members of the MAPK family including p38 kinase (p38), extracellular stress-related kinase 1/2 (ERK), and stress-activated protein kinase/c-Jun N-terminal kinase (JNK) (Su 2002). The MAPK family plays important roles in the regulation of cell death and proliferation in response to various cellular stresses. It was reported that D-GalN activates MAPKs (Nishioka et al. 2006).

Therefore, we investigated the TLR4/CD14 pathway, NF-κB, and MAPKs to clarify the mechanism of Biobran's protective effects against D-GalN-induced hepatitis (Zheng et al. 2012b). Wistar rats were injected intraperitoneally with either Biobran or the low molecular weight Biobran fraction. Then, rats were administered D-GalN at a dose of 400 mg/kg 1 h after the initial treatment.

Serum transaminase activity (ALT and AST) was significantly higher after GalN treatment. However, Biobran and the low molecular weight Biobran fraction strongly suppressed these hepatitis parameters. The low molecular weight Biobran fraction significantly attenuated the increase in serum transaminase activity in a dose-dependent manner ($p < 0.05$) (Zheng et al. 2012b). Next, we focused on the hepatoprotective mechanism of the low molecular weight Biobran fraction. At 8 h after D-GalN treatment, liver CD14 mRNA expression levels were significantly higher than those in the normal (non-D-GalN-treated) group. However, the low molecular weight Biobran fraction pre-treatment group showed strong suppression of CD14 mRNA expression in the liver compared with the control (D-GalN-treated) group. We also measured the liver TLR4 mRNA expression levels in the normal, D-GalN-treated (control), and low molecular weight Biobran fraction-treated groups. There were no significant differences in liver TLR4 mRNA expression levels among the three groups. However, TLR4 mRNA expression showed a similar trend to that of CD14 mRNA expression among the three groups (Zheng et al. 2012b).

NF-κB translocates to the nucleus via phosphorylation and degradation of IκBα. We examined the effect of the low molecular weight Biobran fraction on IκBα degradation, and we found that fraction strongly inhibited D-GalN-induced IκBα degradation 8 h after D-GalN treatment. When we studied the effect on the MAPK signaling pathways, we found that pre-treatment with the low molecular weight Biobran fraction significantly inhibited D-GalN-activated phosphorylation of JNK in the liver (Zheng et al. 2012b). These findings showed that the suppressive effect of Biobran on D-GalN-induced liver injury is related to the inhibition of NF-κB, MAPK, and CD14 expression (Fig. 11.1).

11.5 Effect of Biobran on Hepatitis C Virus Patients

Plasma IL-18 was significantly increased in patients with liver injury that was caused by HCV infection (Murata et al. 2005; Vecchiet et al. 2005). Biobran suppressed D-GalN hepatitis and the IL-18 concentration (Zheng et al. 2012a), so it might also suppress HCV infection.

Salama et al. reported that Biobran suppresses the viremia level in patients with chronic HCV infection (Salama et al. 2016). In a non-inferiority clinical trial, two groups of chronic HCV patients ($n = 37$) were randomized to receive either pegylated interferon (IFN, 180 μg, subcutaneously weekly) plus ribavirin (1200 mg for over 75 kg BW or 1000 mg for under 75 kg) as a standard treatment ($n = 21$) or Biobran (1 g/day, $n = 16$) for 3 months (Salama et al. 2016). They examined viremia, liver enzyme levels, serum IFN-γ, and toxicity before and 3 months after treatment. Viral load was examined using a quantitative polymerase chain reaction test. Post-treatment, the viral load in both groups was reduced to a similar extent. Patients who received pegylated IFN plus ribavirin showed a significantly decreased viral load compared with the baseline value (median baseline, 300,000 IU/mL; median after 3 months, 16 IU/mL). Patients who received Biobran also had a significantly reduced viral load compared with the baseline value (median

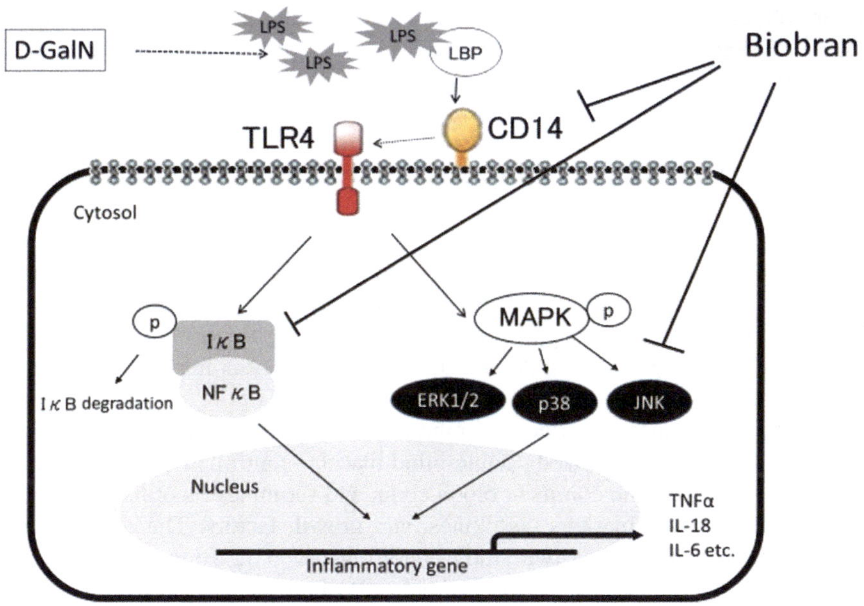

Fig. 11.1 The suppressive effect of Biobran on D-GalN-induced liver injury

baseline, 224,000 IU/mL; median after 3 months, 70,150 IU/mL) (Salama et al. 2016). Patients in both groups showed a significant reduction in the viral load relative to the baseline value ($P < 0.05$). Patients who received pegylated IFN plus ribavirin showed significantly decreased liver enzyme (ALT) levels compared with the baseline value (mean ± standard deviation [SD] at baseline, 59.7 ± 43.3 U/L; after 3 months, 42.8 ± 24.9 U/L, P < 0.05). Patients who received Biobran showed a 21.3% increase in ALT levels and an 11.0% increase in AST levels compared with the baseline values, but this difference was not statistically significant. However, treatment with Biobran caused a twofold ($P < 0.001$) increase of IFN-γ level after 3 months (mean ± SD at baseline, 16.1 ± 1.7 pg/mL; after 3 months, 34.4 ± 19.8 pg/mL) (Salama et al. 2016). Some studies reported that IFN-γ is a potent inhibitor of viral replication (Frese et al. 2002). Moreover, Biobran also modulates immune cells such as CD4+ and CD8+ T cells and NK cells, which play major role in antiviral infection (Ghoneum and Abedi 2004; Ghoneum and Agrawal 2014). The authors speculated that Biobran might act as a therapeutic vaccine by boosting the host protective cell-mediated immune responses against HCV (Salama et al. 2016).

Next, Salama et al. evaluated the toxicity of pegylated IFN plus ribavirin and Biobran treatment using a questionnaire, physicians' observations, and laboratory test results. They reported that patients who received pegylated IFN plus ribavirin showed adverse events including mild fatigue (47.6%), fever (95.2%), digestive disorder (95.2%), hepatomegaly (71.4%), weight loss (47.6%), dry cough, anemia, and thrombocytopenia, while patients who received Biobran showed no such side effects (0%) except for hepatomegaly (68.8%) and reported good health (Salama et al. 2016).

11.6 Effect of Biobran on Nonalcoholic Fatty Liver Disease Patients

NAFLD is a spectrum of diseases that are characterized by fat accumulation in the liver. The incidence and prevalence of NAFLD are increasing worldwide. There is a paucity of available treatment approaches besides reducing the fat content in the liver via weight loss (Schwenger and Allard 2014). Therefore, it is important to explore nutritional interventions.

Lewis et al. examined the effect of Biobran on biomarkers in adults ($n = 23$) with NAFLD in a 90-day randomized double-blind placebo-controlled trial (Lewis et al. 2018). They measured the complete blood count and serum levels of liver enzymes, lipids, oxidative stress markers, cytokines, and growth factors. The patients were randomly assigned to one of two study conditions ($n = 12$ Biobran and $n = 11$ placebo), and they consumed 1 g/day of either Biobran or the control compound, respectively, for 90 days. There were no adverse effects under these experimental conditions. The level of the hepatic enzyme alkaline phosphatase (ALP) significantly decreased in the Biobran group compared with placebo ($p < 0.05$). An increasing ALP level suggests that there is liver damage, and it is related to steatosis and fibrosis (Khodadoostan et al. 2016).

The percent monocytes and percent eosinophils increased in the Biobran group compared with the placebo. The increase in the percentage of both eosinophils and monocytes in the Biobran group suggests that there is an immunomodulatory response. A short-term mild inflammatory response could be beneficial to protect hepatocytes from damage and to achieve homeostasis (Lewis et al. 2018).

IFN-γ levels also increased in the Biobran group compared with placebo. Although not statistically significant, IL-18 decreased from 446 pg/mL at baseline to 221 pg/mL at 90 days in the Biobran group, whereas IL-18 levels in the placebo group slightly increased from baseline (256 pg/mL) to 90 days (263 pg/mL) (Lewis et al. 2018).

Other improvements were noted for platelets, neutrophils, the neutrophil-to-lymphocyte ratio, γ-glutamyl transferase, and 4-hydroxynonenal (Lewis et al. 2018). These findings imply that Biobran improves inflammation, liver function, and oxidative stress in patients with NAFLD. Treatment of NAFLD patients is limited by conventionally supplied medicine. Moreover, there is no treatment other than reducing the fat in the liver. Biobran seems to have beneficial effects on several biomarkers in people with NAFLD.

11.7 Conclusion

In humans, Biobran had a positive effect on hepatitis C and NAFLD under the experimental conditions that were described in this chapter. In animal experiments, Biobran was observed to prevent D-GalN-induced hepatitis. Inhibition of IL-18 seems to be important because serum IL-18 concentrations increase in various diseases such as animal models of atopic dermatitis and bronchial asthma and in patients with HCV (Murata et al. 2005; Tanaka et al. 2001; Lee et al. 2006).

More clinical and basic research on Biobran is required in the future to clarify its positive effects and mechanisms of action.

References

Akira S, Hemmi H (2003) Recognition of pathogen-associated molecular patterns by TLR family. Immunol Lett 85:85–95

Daizo A, Egashira Y, Sanada H (2005) Suppressive effect of corn bran hemicellulose on liver injury induced by D-galactosamine in rats. Nutrition 21:1044–1051

Daizo A, Egashira Y, Sanada H (2006) Effects of dietary corn bran hemicellulose and neomycin on hepatic caspase-3 activity and glycoprotein concentration in rats treated with or without D-galactosamine. J Nutr Sci Vitaminol (Tokyo) 52:96–104

Decker K, Keppler D (1974) Galactosamine hepatitis: key role of the nucleotide deficiency period in the pathogenesis of cell injury and cell death. Rev Physiol Biochem Pharmacol (71):77–106

Finotto S, Siebler J, Hausding M, Schipp M, Wirtz S, Klein S et al (2004) Severe hepatic injury in interleukin 18 (IL-18) transgenic mice: a key role for IL-18 in regulating hepatocyte apoptosis in vivo. Gut 53:392–400

Frese M, Schwärzle V, Barth K, Krieger N, Lohmann V, Mihm S et al (2002) Interferon-gamma inhibits replication of subgenomic and genomic hepatitis C virus RNAs. Hepatology 35:694–703

Galanos C, Freudenberg MA, Reutter W (1979) Galactosamine-induced sensitization to the lethal effects of endotoxin. Proc Natl Acad Sci U S A 76:5939–5943

Ghoneum M, Abedi S (2004) Enhancement of natural killer cell activity of aged mice by modified arabinoxylan rice bran (MGN-3/Biobran). J Pharm Pharmacol 56:1581–1588

Ghoneum M, Agrawal S (2014) MGN-3/Biobran enhances generation of cytotoxic CD8+ T cells via upregulation of DEC-205 expression on dendritic cells. Int J Immunopathol Pharmacol 27: 523–530

Keppler D, Lesch R, Reutter W, Decker K (1968) Experimental hepatitis induced by D-galactosamine. Exp Mol Pathol 9:279–290

Keppler DO, Rudigier JF, Bischoff E, Decker KF (1970) The trapping of uridine phosphates by D-galactosamine, D-glucosamine, and 2-deoxy-D-galactose. A study on the mechanism of galactosamine hepatitis. Eur J Biochem 17:246–253

Khodadoostan M, Shariatifar B, Motamedi N, Abdolahi H (2016) Comparison of liver enzymes level and sonographic findings value with liver biopsy findings in nonalcoholic fatty liver disease patients. Adv Biomed Res 5:40

Komano T, Egashira Y, Sanada H (2008) L-Gln and L-Ser suppress the D-galactosamine-induced IL-18 expression and hepatitis. Biochem Biophys Res Commun 372:688–690

Lee KS, Kim SR, Park SJ, Min KH, Lee KY, Jin SM et al (2006) Antioxidant down-regulates interleukin-18 expression in asthma. Mol Pharmacol 70:1184–1193

Lewis JE, Atlas SE, Higuera OL, Fiallo A, Rasul A, Farooqi A et al (2018) The effect of a hydrolyzed polysaccharide dietary supplement on biomarkers in adults with nonalcoholic fatty liver disease. Evid Based Complement Alternat Med 2018:1751583

Lu J, Ren D-F, Wang J-Z, Sanada H, Egashira Y (2010) Protection by dietary Spirulina platensis against D-galactosamine- and acetaminophen-induced liver injuries. Br J Nutr 103:1573–1576
Mitchell JR, Jollow DJ, Potter WZ, Davis DC, Gillette JR, Brodie BB (1973) Acetaminophen-induced hepatic necrosis. I. Role of drug metabolism. J Pharmacol Exp Ther 187:185–194
Murata K, Yamamoto N, Kawakita T, Saito Y, Yamanaka Y, Sugimoto K et al (2005) Up-regulation of IL-18 by interferon alpha-2b/ribavirin combination therapy induces an anti-viral effect in patients with chronic hepatitis C. Hepato-Gastroenterology 52:547–551
Nishioka H, Kishioka T, Iida C, Fujii K, Ichi I, Kojo S (2006) Activation of mitogen activated protein kinase (MAPK) during D-galactosamine intoxication in the rat liver. Bioorg Med Chem Lett 16:3019–3022
Noaman E, Badr El-Din NK, Bibars MA, Abou Mossallam AA, Ghoneum M (2008) Antioxidant potential by arabinoxylan rice bran, MGN-3/biobran, represents a mechanism for its oncostatic effect against murine solid Ehrlich carcinoma. Cancer Lett 268:348–359
Peng Y, Gong J-P, Liu C-A, Li X-H, Gan L, Li S-B (2004) Expression of toll-like receptor 4 and MD-2 gene and protein in Kupffer cells after ischemia-reperfusion in rat liver graft. World J Gastroenterol 10:2890–2893
Salama H, Medhat E, Shaheen M, Zekri A-RN, Darwish T, Ghoneum M (2016) Arabinoxylan rice bran (Biobran) suppresses the viremia level in patients with chronic HCV infection: a randomized trial. Int J Immunopathol Pharmacol 29:647–653
Sanada H, Egashira Y (2009) Hepatic injury and luminacoid/dietary fiber. J Japanese Assoc Diet Fiber Res 13:1–10
Schwabe RF, Seki E, Brenner DA (2006) Toll-like receptor signaling in the liver. Gastroenterology 130:1886–1900
Schwenger KJP, Allard JP (2014) Clinical approaches to non-alcoholic fatty liver disease. World J Gastroenterol 20:1712–1723
Stachlewitz RF, Seabra V, Bradford B, Bradham CA, Rusyn I, Germolec D et al (1999) Glycine and uridine prevent D-galactosamine hepatotoxicity in the rat: role of Kupffer cells. Hepatology 29: 737–745
Su GL (2002) Lipopolysaccharides in liver injury: molecular mechanisms of Kupffer cell activation. Am J Physiol Liver Physiol 283:G256–G265
Tanaka T, Tsutsui H, Yoshimoto T, Kotani M, Matsumoto M, Fujita A et al (2001) Interleukin-18 is elevated in the sera from patients with atopic dermatitis and from atopic dermatitis model mice, NC/Nga. Int Arch Allergy Immunol 125:236–240
Tsutsui H, Matsui K, Okamura H, Nakanishi K (2000) Pathophysiological roles of interleukin-18 in inflammatory liver diseases. Immunol Rev 174:192–209
Tsutsui H, Adachi K, Seki E, Nakanishi K (2003) Cytokine-induced inflammatory liver injuries. Curr Mol Med 3:545–559
Vecchiet J, Falasca K, Cacciatore P, Zingariello P, Dalessandro M, Marinopiccoli M et al (2005) Association between plasma interleukin-18 levels and liver injury in chronic hepatitis C virus infection and non-alcoholic fatty liver disease. Ann Clin Lab Sci 35:415–422
Wang B, Chewchuang C, Egashira Y, Ohta T, Sanada H (1995) Effects of oligosaccharides on galactosamine hepatitis in rats. Nippon Eiyo Shokuryo Gakkaishi 48:181–187
Wang B, Egashira Y, Ohta T, Sanada H (1998) Effect of indigestible oligosaccharides on the hepatotoxic action of D-galactosamine in rats. Biosci Biotechnol Biochem 62:1504–1509
Zheng S, Sanada H, Dohi H, Hirai S, Egashira Y (2012a) Suppressive effect of modified arabinoxylan from rice bran (MGN-3) on D-galactosamine-induced IL-18 expression and hepatitis in rats. Biosci Biotechnol Biochem 76:942–946
Zheng S, Sugita S, Hirai S, Egashira Y (2012b) Protective effect of low molecular fraction of MGN-3, a modified arabinoxylan from rice bran, on acute liver injury by inhibition of NF-κB and JNK/MAPK expression. Int Immunopharmacol 14:764–769

Additional Potential Therapeutic Applications for Rice Bran Arabinoxylan Compound

12

Peter S. Micalos, Sok Cheon Pak, and Soo Liang Ooi

Abstract

This chapter highlights the research literature on using rice bran arabinoxylan compound (RBAC) as a nutraceutical and functional food for a range of acute and chronic conditions. RBAC has shown potential for supporting the liver, particularly in fatty liver disease, which involves an accumulation of fat in the parenchymal cells of the liver. Chronic fatigue syndrome (CFS) is a persistent relapsing fatigue not alleviated by rest and exacerbated by moderate exercise. Research suggests that RBAC may support persons with CFS. Common colds and influenza are the most common diseases in humans. Studies on RBAC show beneficial effects in reducing the physical stress associated with acute respiratory tract infections and reveals prophylactic effects. Diabetes mellitus (DM) is a group of disorders characterised by hyperglycaemia resulting from insulin resistance, inadequate insulin secretion, or excessive glucagon secretion. In animal-based studies, RBAC reveals therapeutic potential for DM through multiple pathways. Irritable bowel syndrome (IBS) involves a disordered communication between the gut and brain, resulting in disturbances in motility, visceral hypersensitivity, and altered central nervous system processing. Previous research indicates that the administration of RBAC improves IBS symptoms, which may be associated with the compound's anti-inflammatory and immune-modulatory effects. Rheumatoid arthritis (RA) is a progressive inflammatory autoimmune disease associated with articular and systemic effects. Case studies of RBAC administration in chronic rheumatism have shown improvements in pain, quality of life, and serological assessments. Although the available evidence indicates the therapeutic

P. S. Micalos · S. C. Pak (✉) · S. L. Ooi
School of Dentistry and Medical Sciences, Charles Sturt University, Bathurst, NSW, Australia
e-mail: spak@csu.edu.au

S. C. Pak et al. (eds.), *Modified Rice Bran Arabinoxylan*,
https://doi.org/10.1007/978-981-19-5735-2_12

benefits of RBAC in these disorders, further research is required to explain the mechanisms for altering the pathophysiology of the disease pathways.

Keywords

Fatty liver disease · Chronic fatigue syndrome · Common cold · Diabetes · Irritable bowel syndrome · Rheumatoid arthritis

12.1 Introduction

The bran layer of rice grain is a source of many nutrients, phytochemicals, and antioxidants (Ooi et al. 2021). A primary constituent in the bran layer is arabinoxylan, a non-starch polysaccharide. Arabinoxylan contains cross-links in the side chains making it resistant to extraction by water (Mendez-Encinas et al. 2018). Extraction methods using enzymes and alkali solutions have enabled the availability of low molecular weight arabinoxylans. A prime example is a modified arabinoxylan product treated with the *Lentinus edodes* mycelial enzyme known as rice bran arabinoxylan compound (RBAC). RBAC is now gaining attention for its health-promoting properties as a nutraceutical and functional food (Ooi et al. 2021; Schupfer et al. 2021). This chapter highlights the peer-reviewed scientific literature on the use of RBAC for fatty liver disease, chronic fatigue syndrome, the common cold, diabetes, irritable bowel syndrome, and rheumatoid arthritis.

12.2 Fatty Liver Disease

Fatty liver disease (FLD) involves an accumulation of fat in the parenchymal cells of the liver, referred to as hepatosteatosis (Toshikuni et al. 2014). FLD may ensue in individuals through chronic alcohol abuse (Schwartz and Reinus 2012). However, nonalcoholic FLD (NAFLD) is commonly associated with metabolic syndrome, obesity, diabetes, and hyperlipidaemia (Antunes et al. 2021; Chalasani et al. 2012). NAFLD is a serious health problem worldwide, affecting 20–30% of the population in Western countries (Bellentani et al. 2010).

The pathological presentation of NAFLD varies from simple hepatic steatosis to steatohepatitis, liver cirrhosis, and hepatocellular carcinoma (Rinella 2015). Although most cases of FLD experience simple hepatic steatosis, some will develop steatohepatitis, with a small percentage of individuals progressing to more severe liver fibrosis and cirrhosis (Toshikuni et al. 2014). The pathophysiology is complex, with multiple signals from visceral adipose tissue disrupting lipid and glucose metabolism. This leads to an accumulation of fat in hepatic tissues and manifests a proinflammatory environment which triggers injury to the liver and other tissues (Rinella 2015). In some patients, continued oxidative stress and lipotoxicity contributes to liver damage, fibrosis, and hepatocellular cancer.

There is a paucity of effective treatments for the management of FLD. Conventional medicine has provided limited efficacious therapy for patients (Lombardi et al. 2017). Lifestyle-mediated weight loss in combination with exercise remains the primary mode of treatment (Parnell et al. 2012). RBAC acting as a functional food and prebiotic has shown potential for supporting the liver.

In an experimental animal study, D-galactosamine was used to induce acute hepatitis to investigate the protective effects of RBAC and a low molecular weight fraction isolated from RBAC (LMW) (Zheng et al. 2012). Serum levels of alanine and aspartate amino transferases (ALT and AST) were assessed after LMW or RBAC administration to determine liver injury, compared to control. The results showed attenuation of serums levels of ALT and AST in both the RBAC- and LMW-treated animals ($P < 0.05$). LMW also annulled the degradation of inhibitor κB kinase induced by D-galactosamine ($P < 0.05$). Moreover, LMW suppressed CD14 mRNA expression and reduced the activation of mitogen-activated protein kinases such as stress-activated protein kinase/c-Jun N-terminal kinase. These results suggest the hepato-protective effects of RBAC and the LMW fraction isolated from RBAC.

The effect of RBAC on biomarkers in adults with NAFLD was investigated by Lewis et al. (2018). This research involved a double-blind design and included 23 adults on stable NAFLD medication. Participants were randomly assigned to the RBAC ($n = 12$) and placebo ($n = 11$) groups and consumed 1 g/day of RBAC and the control compound, respectively, for 90 days. Biomarkers assessed included the complete blood count, serum levels of liver enzymes, lipids, oxidative stress markers, and cytokines. The results showed that the level of hepatic enzyme alkaline phosphatase (ALP) significantly decreased in the RBAC group ($P = 0.02$) compared to the placebo group. A high level of ALP level suggests liver damage and is associated with steatosis and fibrosis. Also, the percentages of monocytes and eosinophils were shown to be significantly increased in the RBAC group compared to the control group (17.9%, $P = 0.02$; 30.6%, $P < 0.01$, respectively). Other improvements in biomarkers of the RBAC group compared to control included platelets, neutrophil percentages, neutrophil-lymphocyte ratio, γ-glutamyl transferase, and 4-hydroxynonenal. This study demonstrated that RBAC conferred several beneficial effects in participants with NAFLD with no adverse effects under the experimental conditions (Lewis et al. 2018).

12.3 Chronic Fatigue Syndrome

Chronic fatigue syndrome (CFS) is a complex debilitating disease of increasing social and economic importance. The condition is characterised by persistent relapsing fatigue of greater than 6 months that is not alleviated by rest and is exacerbated by moderate exercise (Krupp et al. 1991; Fukuda et al. 1994). Previous phenomenological research suggests that a discrete fatigue syndrome is distinguished from anxiety and depression (Hickie et al. 1999). Persons with CFS often experience disturbed sleep, cognitive difficulties, and muscle weakness (Petrovics et al. 2016).

Although women are statistically more susceptible than men, the disease has also been diagnosed in children and adolescents, as well as across a wide range of ethnic groups (Jordan et al. 1998). Despite the fact that abnormalities are shown across several domains such as immunological, brain architecture and function, neuroendocrine, and virological, the aetiology of CFS remains elusive (Afari and Buchwald 2003).

CFS is a controversial disorder in relation to its clinical definition and aetiopathogenesis (Cho et al. 2006). A meta-analysis (Johnston et al. 2013) showed the pooled prevalence of self-reported CFS at 3.28% (95% CI: 2.24–4.33). Moreover, chronic fatigue often presents in cancer patients. Clinicians have applied a wide range of pharmacological treatments for various aspects of CFS. However, a previous review on pharmacological intervention for CFS revealed inconclusive or insufficient evidence for the effects of these treatments (Afari and Buchwald 2003).

In a combination intervention for CFS, RBAC supplement and oncothermia was evaluated in cancer patients suffering from CFS due to chemotherapy (Petrovics et al. 2016). Oncothermia involves increased temperature applied to malignant tumours. The study spanned over 6 months and involved 30 cancer patients in the RBAC+oncothermia group and 30 participants in the control group under routine care. Oncothermia was applied once per week over 15 weeks, and 1 g of RBAC was required to be taken three times per day over 24 weeks. The results showed that the symptoms of fatigue as measured by the Chalder fatigue questionnaire (CFQ) reduced significantly after the combined treatment ($P < 0.01$), whereas CFQ scores of the control group did not change significantly. Moreover, the average Patient Global Impression of Change (PGIC) after the treatment was 2.1 ± 0.5 ('much improved') which shows the patients perceived that the therapy could help to reduce CFS symptoms. In the non-treatment group, the PGIC score was 4.3 ± 0.9 ('no changes') (Petrovics et al. 2016). Based on these findings, the combination of RBAC and oncothermia may support the symptomatic treatment of CFS in cancer patients.

In a descriptive study by Kenyon (2001) on RBAC use in patients with CFS, ten participants consumed RBAC three times per day for 2 months. Participants completed the CFQ and a visual analogue scale for fatigue before and after the 2 months of RBAC administration. The results showed that four patients clearly improved, one patient withdrew from the study, two patients became worse, and three patients showed no change. From the patient history, some patients showing negative outcomes had experienced exposure to pesticides and laboratory chemicals. It was reported that this may have influenced the results in these patients. Kenyon (2001) concluded that those patients showing improvements with RBAC had a viral CFS aetiology. Moreover, the improvements in CFS symptomology among these patients persisted for approximately 6 weeks after RBAC treatment.

In research by McDermott et al. (2006), the effect of RBAC was investigated in 71 participants with CFS. RBAC was taken by participants at a 2 g dose three times per day over 8 weeks or a placebo equivalent. Sixty-four participants completed the trial, with both the RBAC and placebo groups showing a marked improvement in symptoms over the study duration with no significant difference between the groups.

However, the RBAC group's CFQ score (physical scale) was 0.3 lower (95% CI: 2.6 to 3.2) than the placebo group, although this was not statistically significant. The study hypothesised that a potential mechanism for RBAC on CFS is the increased natural killer (NK) cell activity. Previous research has shown that CFS is associated with low NK cell activity and that RBAC can increase NK cell activity (Pérez-Martínez et al. 2015). However, the research by McDermott et al. (2006) did not measure NK cell activity.

12.4 Common Cold

The most common diseases in humans are acute upper respiratory tract infections, including the common cold and influenza (flu), which are syndromes caused by viruses. There is substantial overlap in the aetiology and symptoms of common cold and flu (Eccles 2005). For example, cold viruses such as respiratory syncytial virus are responsible for many flulike illnesses, while influenza viruses account for 5–15% of colds (Zambon et al. 2001). Approximately 30–50% of all common colds are caused by rhinoviruses, and 10–15% are caused by coronaviruses (Heikkinen and Järvinen 2003).

In the context of experimental colds, the common cold syndrome has been defined as a short, mild illness with early symptoms of headache, sneezing, chilliness, and sore throat and later symptoms of nasal discharge, nasal obstruction, cough, and malaise (Eccles 2005; Jackson et al. 1958). Influenza syndrome usually has a sudden onset and is typified by fever, headache, cough, sore throat, myalgia, nasal congestion, weakness, and loss of appetite (Monto et al. 2000).

Understanding the pathogenic events that underly the common cold is derived from studies involving volunteers infected with rhinoviruses (Winther et al. 1986). Rhinovirus infection begins when the virus deposits in the nasal mucosa or the eye and travels to the posterior nasopharynx. Most rhinoviruses gain entry into epithelial cells via specific receptors such as intercellular adhesion molecule-1. Once inside the cell, the virus rapidly replicates and is detectible within 8–10 h following intranasal inoculation (Heikkinen and Järvinen 2003). Shedding of the virus, when viral particles exit while talking or eating, for example, peaks on the second day after intranasal inoculation and remains detectible for up to 3 weeks after infection.

The deterioration in the function of the immune system with ageing is referred to as immunosenescence (Gruver et al. 2007). Due to reduced immune function, the elderly are more susceptible to infection and increased risk of complications and hospitalisations (Laue et al. 2021). The immune response to vaccination in the elderly has been shown to be weaker compared to younger adults. To protect the elderly from infectious diseases, novel strategies such as nutritional interventions that boost the immune response might improve health and reduce the risk of disease (Elsaid et al. 2020).

Oral administration of RBAC to prevent the common cold was researched in 50 elderly persons aged 70–95 years (Maeda et al. 2004). The research design involved a double-blind cross-over study using water-soluble rice bran (RB) as the control. Thirty-six participants completed the trial, with no withdrawals due to any side effects of the experimental foods. The results showed that the average duration of cold symptoms was 2.6 days for RB, and for the RBAC it was 1.2 days. Additionally, the total symptom score for the RB treatment group was three times higher than that for the RBAC treatment group. The study concluded that RBAC was beneficial in reducing the physical stress associated with acute respiratory tract infection.

In another study by Elsaid et al. (2021), dietary supplementation with RBAC on the incidence of influenza-like illness was investigated in elderly participants. The research design was a double-blind, placebo-controlled clinical trial with 80 healthy older adults over 55 years old, 40 males and 40 females, who received either a placebo or RBAC (500 mg/day) for 3 months. The incidence of influenza-like illness was confirmed clinically according to the WHO case definition criteria. Results showed that among the RBAC group, the incidence rate and incidence density of influenza-like illness was 5.0% and 0.57 cases per 1000 person-days, compared to 22.5% and 2.95 cases per 1000 person-days in the placebo group. Additional assessment in six participants among the RBAC group revealed significantly enhanced NK cell activity compared to basal levels and to another six participants in the placebo group. Also, several viral detection and antiviral responses were significantly upregulated in the RBAC group. These results suggest that RBAC shows prophylactic effects against a broad spectrum of respiratory viral infections that warrants further investigation.

12.5 Diabetes

Diabetes mellitus (DM) is a group of disorders characterised by hyperglycaemia resulting from insulin resistance, inadequate insulin secretion, or excessive glucagon secretion (Alam et al. 2014). Diabetes can lead to a range of complications involving microvascular, macrovascular, and neuropathic disorders. Treatment for DM is based on aetiopathology. Most commonly, DM is subdivided into type 1 and type 2 (Blair 2016). Type 1 DM is an autoimmune disorder and ensues when ~90% of pancreatic β cells are destroyed. The more common type 2 DM accounts for 90–95% of cases and is characterised by progressively impaired glucose regulation due to a combination of dysfunctional pancreatic β cells and insulin resistance (Alam et al. 2014). Furthermore, the underlying pathophysiological mechanisms of type 2 DM involve the generation of reactive oxygen species and reactive nitrogen species via activation of advanced glycation end-products, polyol flux, hexosamine, and protein kinase C pathways (Folli et al. 2011; Hameed et al. 2015) that leads to cell stress. As a result, this progresses to the development of insulin resistance, cell dysfunction, and impaired glucose tolerance. Several signalling proteins involved in inflammation such as TNF-α, IL-1β, and interferon-γ are also upregulated, leading to insulin resistance and hyperglycaemia (Rachana et al. 2015).

In a review article by Saji et al. (2019), the effect of rice bran-derived bioactive compounds in type 2 DM was highlighted. These compounds, such as polyphenols, tocotrienol, and oryzanol, have been shown to improve precursor pathways associated with type 2 DM, including hyperglycaemia, hypertension, and hyperlipidaemia. In research by Alauddin et al. (2016) on stroke-prone hypertensive rats, 4-week treatment with fermented rice bran showed several favourable outcomes such as reduced hypertension, insulin, glucose, and total cholesterol. These results imply that rice bran extract such as RBAC may offer therapeutic potential for diabetes through multiple pathways.

At present, there are no published human research trials showing the potential therapeutic effects of RBAC for diabetic patients. However, in an animal research trial by Ohara et al. (2002), the effect of RBAC on glucose tolerance in adult rats was investigated. Diabetes in the experimental animals was induced by streptozotocin (STZ), an antibiotic that causes pancreatic islet β-cell destruction. The experimental procedure included a dietary intervention consisting of 1.7% cellulose or 1.7% cellulose plus 1% RBAC for 60 days. Glucose tolerance testing was performed after 20 h of fasting on day 58. The results showed the diabetic rats fed with RBAC had significantly lower glucose levels ($P < 0.05$) at 30 min after being fed with glucose (2 g/kg body mass) compared to the control diet. Additional testing also revealed a lower cholesterol level in the RBAC fed rats compared to the control animals. These results suggest that supplementation with RBAC attenuates blood glucose levels as well as lipid metabolism in diabetic rats.

Ohara et al. (2000) also investigated the effect of RBAC on taste preference in STZ-induced diabetic rats. Control rats were administered 0.5% sodium alginate, and the experimental rats were administered RBAC at 0.5 g/kg body mass. A two-bottle choice preference test was performed with deionised water (DW) and a flavoured solution. Rats were divided into four groups of citric acid (sour) + DW, sodium saccharin (sweet) + DW, monosodium glutamate (savoury) + DW, or quinine (bitter) + DW. Results showed that the intake of water was reduced in the RBAC rats, which suggests that polyuria induced by STZ was improved. Serum triglycerides and total cholesterol decreased with the administration of RBAC, although serum insulin and glucose remained low and high, respectively. Diabetic rats showed significant aversion to citric acid (sour) and quinine (bitterness) when compared with control rats. The study concluded that RBAC can be useful as a dietary supplement for the treatment of diabetes.

12.6 Irritable Bowel Syndrome

Irritable bowel syndrome (IBS) is a functional gastrointestinal disorder that affects between 5% and 10% of healthy individuals and, in most people, runs a relapsing and remitting course (Ford et al. 2020). The pathophysiology of IBS is incompletely understood. However, it has been shown that there is disordered communication between the gut and brain, resulting in disturbances in motility, visceral hypersensitivity, and altered central nervous system processing. Symptoms include abdominal pain with a change in stool form or frequency. There are three major subtypes of IBS. IBS-D is associated primarily with diarrhoea, IBS-C is affected with constipation, and the third subtype is related to mixed constipation and diarrhoea symptoms (Bruta et al. 2021). There is also evidence showing low-grade mucosal inflammation and/or immune dysfunction in the lower gastrointestinal tract (Barbara et al. 2004). Treatment of IBS is often targeted towards the predominant symptom that the patient experiences (Talley et al. 2015). Pharmacological interventions such as central modulators or 5-HT3 receptor antagonists may be used for more severe cases. However, treatments are often not sufficiently effective and the disorder results in a considerable adverse impact on the quality of life (QOL).

The therapeutic effects of RBAC supplementation have been previously investigated in diarrhoea-predominant or mixed-type IBS. In research by Kamiya et al. (2014), 40 patients with IBS were randomly assigned to either a RBAC treatment group or a placebo group. The RBAC group consumed 1 g × 2 per day, and the control group consumed a placebo powder that included dietary fibre. IBS symptoms and the therapeutic efficacy were assessed subjectively by the patients after 4 weeks of administration. The study reported that global symptom assessment improved 63.2% in the RBAC group compared to 30% in the placebo group, which was statistically significant ($P < 0.05$). Also, the RBAC group showed a significant reduction in the diarrhoea and constipation score and in the C-reactive protein (CRP) value. In contrast, there were no significant changes observed in the placebo group. These results indicate that the administration of RBAC improved IBS symptoms, which may be associated with the anti-inflammatory and/or immune-modulatory effects of this supplement.

12.7 Rheumatoid Arthritis

Rheumatoid arthritis (RA) is a progressive inflammatory autoimmune disease associated with articular and systemic effects (Choy 2012). The exact cause is unknown, however, an interplay between genetic and environmental factors contributes to the disease process. More than 80% of patients carry a shared epitope of the HLA-DRB1*04 cluster (Smolen et al. 2007). The shared epitope is a five-amino acid sequence which is the most significant genetic risk factor (Fu et al. 2018). A greater risk of RA exists in women compared to men. Other risk factors such as smoking and adverse life events are associated with RA onset (McInnes and Schett 2011). Pharmacological treatment includes drugs that act on the immunoinflammatory pathways in RA, such as disease-modifying antirheumatic drugs and biological agents, although the frequency and degree of responses are limited (Smolen et al. 2007).

The administration of RBAC in chronic rheumatism has been investigated in eight patient cases by Ichihashi (2004). RBAC was administered at 1–3 g/day for 6–12 months to observe changes in subjective symptoms, QOL, and plasma CRP. The results showed three patients responded well to the RBAC supplement. For example, case 1 was a 78-year-old woman who was almost bedridden and presented with severe pain, walking difficulty, and progressive bone destruction. Serological tests showed ++ for RA index, 65 IU/ml for rheumatoid factor (RF), and 2.0 mg/dl for CRP. After 1 week of RBAC treatment, this patient had pain relief in the hands and feet with better sleep. After 1 month, this patient could walk using a walker. After 8 months of RBAC administration, the RA test was negative, RF was reduced to 14 IU/ml, and CRP was decreased to 0.6 mg/dl. Furthermore, three of the eight patients had improvements in subjective symptoms, especially pain and QOL. There were also improvements in serological assessments such as the RA index and CRP. In two of these patients, anti-inflammatory steroid drugs were no longer required, and the dose was reduced in the third patient.

12.8 Conclusion

Previous research advocates the use of RBAC as a functional food to support human health. In NAFLD, RBAC showed decreased hepatic ALP enzyme compared to the control, which suggests a reduced liver damage in the RBAC group. For CFS, several pharmacological treatments have not been effective, however, RBAC combined with oncothermia has been shown to reduce the symptom of fatigue in cancer patients with CFS. In the common cold, RBAC was shown to reduce the incidence rate and density of influenza-like illness, potentially through enhanced NK cell activity. In type 2 diabetes, RBAC may show therapeutic potential through several bioactive compounds such as polyphenols, tocotrienol, and oryzanol. For IBS, global symptom assessment improved with RBAC supplementation. In RA, case studies on the use of RBAC reveal improvements in walking capacity, pain scores, and serological markers such as the RA index and CRP. Potential underlying mechanisms for RBAC influencing the disease process are through its bioactive compounds showing anti-inflammatory and/or immune-modulatory effects. Although there is substantial evidence indicating the use of RBAC as a complementary therapy, further research is required to explicate the mechanisms for altering the pathophysiology of disease pathways.

References

Afari N, Buchwald D (2003) Chronic fatigue syndrome: a review. Am J Psychiatry 160:221–236

Alam U, Asghar O, Azmi S, Malik RA (2014) General aspects of diabetes mellitus. Handb Clin Neurol 126:211–222

Alauddin M, Shirakawa H, Koseki T, Kijima N, Ardiansyah, Budijanto S et al (2016) Fermented rice bran supplementation mitigates metabolic syndrome in stroke-prone spontaneously hypertensive rats. BMC Complement Altern Med 16:442

Antunes C, Azadfard M, Hoilat GJ, Gupta M (2021) Fatty liver. In: StatPearls [internet]. StatPearls Publishing, Treasure Island, FL. https://www.ncbi.nlm.nih.gov/books/NBK441992/

Barbara G, Stanghellini V, De Giorgio R, Cremon C, Cottrell GS, Santini D et al (2004) Activated mast cells in proximity to colonic nerves correlate with abdominal pain in irritable bowel syndrome. Gastroenterology 126:693–702

Bellentani S, Scaglioni F, Marino M, Bedogni G (2010) Epidemiology of non-alcoholic fatty liver disease. Dig Dis 28:155–161

Blair M (2016) Diabetes mellitus review. Urol Nurs 36:27–36

Bruta K, Vanshika, Bhasin K, Bhawana (2021) The role of serotonin and diet in the prevalence of irritable bowel syndrome: a systematic review. Transl Med Commun 6:1

Chalasani N, Younossi Z, Lavine JE, Diehl AM, Brunt EM, Cusi K et al (2012) The diagnosis and management of non-alcoholic fatty liver disease: practice guideline by the American Association for the Study of Liver Diseases, American College of Gastroenterology, and the American Gastroenterological Association. Hepatology 55:2005–2023

Cho HJ, Skowera A, Cleare A, Wessely S (2006) Chronic fatigue syndrome: an update focusing on phenomenology and pathophysiology. Curr Opin Psychiatry 19:67–73

Choy E (2012) Understanding the dynamics: pathways involved in the pathogenesis of rheumatoid arthritis. Rheumatology 51:v3–v11

Eccles R (2005) Understanding the symptoms of the common cold and influenza. Lancet Infect Dis 5:718–725

Elsaid AF, Fahmi RM, Shaheen M, Ghoneum M (2020) The enhancing effects of Biobran/MGN-3, an arabinoxylan rice bran, on healthy old adults' health-related quality of life: a randomized, double-blind, placebo-controlled clinical trial. Qual Life Res 29:357

Elsaid AF, Agrawal S, Agrawal A, Ghoneum M (2021) Dietary supplementation with Biobran/MGN-3 increases innate resistance and reduces the incidence of influenza-like illnesses in elderly subjects: a randomized, double-blind, placebo-controlled pilot clinical trial. Nutrients 13:4133

Folli F, Corradi D, Fanti P, Davalli A, Paez A, Giaccari A et al (2011) The role of oxidative stress in the pathogenesis of type 2 diabetes mellitus micro- and macrovascular complications: avenues for a mechanistic-based therapeutic approach. Curr Diabetes Rev 7:313–324

Ford AC, Sperber AD, Corsetti M, Camilleri M (2020) Irritable bowel syndrome. Lancet 396:1675–1688

Fu J, Nogueira SV, van Drongelen V, Coit P, Ling S, Rosloniec EF et al (2018) Shared epitope-aryl hydrocarbon receptor crosstalk underlies the mechanism of gene-environment interaction in autoimmune arthritis. Proc Natl Acad Sci U S A 115:4755–4760

Fukuda K, Straus SE, Hickie I, Sharpe MC, Dobbins JG, Komaroff A (1994) The chronic fatigue syndrome: a comprehensive approach to its definition and study. International Chronic Fatigue Syndrome Study Group. Ann Intern Med 121:953–959

Gruver AL, Hudson LL, Sempowski GD (2007) Immunosenescence of ageing. J Pathol 211:144–156

Hameed I, Masoodi SR, Mir SA, Nabi M, Ghazanfar K, Ganai BA (2015) Type 2 diabetes mellitus: from a metabolic disorder to an inflammatory condition. World J Diabetes 6:598–612

Heikkinen T, Järvinen A (2003) The common cold. Lancet 361:51–59

Hickie I, Koschera A, Hadzi-Pavlovic D, Bennett B, Lloyd A (1999) The temporal stability and co-morbidity of prolonged fatigue: a longitudinal study in primary care. Psychol Med 29:855–861

Ichihashi K (2004) Experience with administration of BioBran in patients with chronic rheumatism. Clin Pharmacol Ther 14:459–463

Jackson GG, Dowling HF, Spiesman IG, Boand AV (1958) Transmission of the common cold to volunteers under controlled conditions. I. The common cold as a clinical entity. AMA Arch Intern Med 101:267–278

Johnston S, Brenu EW, Staines D, Marshall-Gradisnik S (2013) The prevalence of chronic fatigue syndrome/ myalgic encephalomyelitis: a meta-analysis. Clin Epidemiol 5:105–110

Jordan KM, Landis DA, Downey MC, Osterman SL, Thurm AE, Jason LA (1998) Chronic fatigue syndrome in children and adolescents: a review. J Adolesc Health 22:4–18

Kamiya T, Shikano M, Tanaka M, Ozeki K, Ebi M, Katano T et al (2014) Therapeutic effects of biobran, modified arabinoxylan rice bran, in improving symptoms of diarrhea predominant or mixed type irritable bowel syndrome: a pilot, randomized controlled study. Evid Based Complement Alternat Med 2014:828137

Kenyon J (2001) A descriptive questionnaire-based study on the use of Biobran (MGN3), in chronic fatigue syndrome. Townsend Lett Dr Patients 220:48–50

Krupp LB, Mendelson WB, Friedman R (1991) An overview of chronic fatigue syndrome. J Clin Psychiatry 52:403–410
Laue C, Stevens Y, van Erp M, Papazova E, Soeth E, Pannenbeckers A et al (2021) Adjuvant effect of orally applied preparations containing non-digestible polysaccharides on influenza vaccination in healthy seniors: a double-blind, randomised, controlled pilot trial. Nutrients 13:2683
Lewis JE, Atlas SE, Higuera OL, Fiallo A, Rasul A, Farooqi A et al (2018) The effect of a hydrolyzed polysaccharide dietary supplement on biomarkers in adults with nonalcoholic fatty liver disease. Evid Based Complement Alternat Med 2018:1751583
Lombardi R, Onali S, Thorburn D, Davidson BR, Gurusamy KS, Tsochatzis E (2017) Pharmacological interventions for non-alcohol related fatty liver disease (NAFLD): an attempted network meta-analysis. Cochrane Database Syst Rev 3:CD011640
Maeda H, Ichihashi K, Fujii T, Omura K, Zhu X, Anazawa M et al (2004) Oral administration of hydrolyzed rice bran prevents the common cold syndrome in the elderly based on its immunomodulatory action. Biofactors 21:185–187
McDermott C, Richards SCM, Thomas PW, Montgomery J, Lewith G (2006) A placebo-controlled, double-blind, randomized controlled trial of a natural killer cell stimulant (BioBran MGN-3) in chronic fatigue syndrome. QJM 99:461–468
McInnes IB, Schett G (2011) The pathogenesis of rheumatoid arthritis. N Engl J Med 365:2205–2219
Mendez-Encinas MA, Carvajal-Millan E, Rascon-Chu A, Astiazaran-Garcia HF, Valencia-Rivera DE (2018) Ferulated arabinoxylans and their gels: functional properties and potential application as antioxidant and anticancer agent. Oxid Med Cell Longev 2018:22
Monto AS, Gravenstein S, Elliott M, Colopy M, Schweinle J (2000) Clinical signs and symptoms predicting influenza infection. Arch Intern Med 160:3243–3247
Ohara I, Tabuchi R, Onai K, Econ MH (2000) Effects of modified rice bran on serum lipids and taste preference in streptozotocin-induced diabetic rats. Nutr Res 20:59–68
Ohara I, Onai K, Maeda H (2002) Modified rice bran improves glucose tolerance in NIDDM adult rats given streptozotocin as neonates. Stud Aichi Gakusen Univ 37:17–23
Ooi SL, Pak SC, Micalos PS, Schupfer E, Lockley C, Park MH et al (2021) The health-promoting properties and clinical applications of rice bran arabinoxylan modified with shiitake mushroom enzyme—a narrative review. Molecules 26:2539
Parnell JA, Raman M, Rioux KP, Reimer RA (2012) The potential role of prebiotic fibre for treatment and management of non-alcoholic fatty liver disease and associated obesity and insulin resistance. Liver Int 32:701–711
Pérez-Martínez A, Valentín J, Fernández L, Hernández-Jiménez E, López-Collazo E, Zerbes P et al (2015) Arabinoxylan rice bran (MGN-3/Biobran) enhances natural killer cell-mediated cytotoxicity against neuroblastoma in vitro and in vivo. Cytotherapy 17:601–612
Petrovics G, Szigeti G, Hamvas S, Máté Á, Betlehem J, Hegyi G (2016) Controlled pilot study for cancer patients suffering from chronic fatigue syndrome due to chemotherapy treated with BioBran (MGN-3-Arabinoxylane) and targeted radiofrequency heat therapy. Eur J Integr Med 8:29–35
Rachana, Thakur S, Basu S (2015) Oxidative stress and diabetes. In: Rani V, Yadav UCS (eds) Free radicals in human health & diseases. Springer, New Delhi, pp 241–257
Rinella ME (2015) Nonalcoholic fatty liver disease: a systematic review. JAMA 313:2263–2273
Saji N, Francis N, Schwarz LJ, Blanchard CL, Santhakumar AB (2019) Rice bran derived bioactive compounds modulate risk factors of cardiovascular disease and type 2 diabetes mellitus: an updated review. Nutrients 11:2736
Schupfer E, Pak SC, Wang S, Micalos PS, Jeffries T, Ooi SL et al (2021) The effects and benefits of arabinoxylans on human gut microbiota – a narrative review. Food Biosci 43:101267
Schwartz JM, Reinus JF (2012) Prevalence and natural history of alcoholic liver disease. Clin Liver Dis 16:659–666
Smolen JS, Aletaha D, Koeller M, Weisman MH, Emery P (2007) New therapies for treatment of rheumatoid arthritis. Lancet 370:1861–1874

Talley NJ, Holtmann G, Walker MM (2015) Therapeutic strategies for functional dyspepsia and irritable bowel syndrome based on pathophysiology. J Gastroenterol 50:601–613
Toshikuni N, Tsutsumi M, Arisawa T (2014) Clinical differences between alcoholic liver disease and nonalcoholic fatty liver disease. World J Gastroenterol 20:8393–8406
Winther B, Gwaltney JMJ, Mygind N, Turner RB, Hendley JO (1986) Sites of rhinovirus recovery after point inoculation of the upper airway. JAMA 256:1763–1767
Zambon MC, Stockton JD, Clewley JP, Fleming DM (2001) Contribution of influenza and respiratory syncytial virus to community cases of influenza-like illness: an observational study. Lancet 358:1410–1416
Zheng S, Sugita S, Hirai S, Egashira Y (2012) Protective effect of low molecular fraction of MGN-3, a modified arabinoxylan from rice bran, on acute liver injury by inhibition of NF-κB and JNK/MAPK expression. Int Immunopharmacol 14:764–769

Index

S. C. Pak et al. (eds.), *Modified Rice Bran Arabinoxylan*,
https://doi.org/10.1007/978-981-19-5735-2

GPSR Compliance

The European Union's (EU) General Product Safety Regulation (GPSR) is a set of rules that requires consumer products to be safe and our obligations to ensure this.

If you have any concerns about our products, you can contact us on ProductSafety@springernature.com

In case Publisher is established outside the EU, the EU authorized representative is:

Springer Nature Customer Service Center GmbH
Europaplatz 3
69115 Heidelberg, Germany

Batch number: 10755034

Printed by Printforce, the Netherlands